Your Over-35 Week-by-Week Pregnancy Guide

Your Over-35 Week-by-Week Pregnancy Guide

All the Answers to All Your Questions
About Pregnancy, Birth, and
Your Developing Baby

M. KELLY SHANAHAN, M.D.

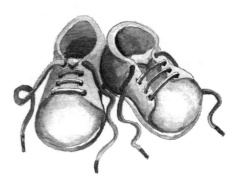

THREE RIVERS PRESS • NEW YORK

Published by Three Rivers Press, New York, New York.
Member of the Crown Publishing Group, a division of Random House, Inc.
www.crownpublishing.com

THREE RIVERS PRESS and the Tugboat design are registered trademarks of Random House, Inc.

Originally published by Prima Publishing, Roseville, California, in 2001.

The information provided in this book is not intended to be a substitute for professional or medical advice. Readers should consult a qualified physician concerning their particular pregnancy. The author and publisher specifically disclaim any liability, loss or risk, personal or otherwise, which is incurred as a result, directly or indirectly, of the use and application of any of the contents of this book.

Illustrations by Steve Larson, M.D., and Mike Fiedler
Interior photos by M. Kelly Shanahan, M.D., Jeff Turney, and Karen Linsley of Image Angels Photography

Printed in the United States of America

Library of Congress Cataloging-in-Publication Data

Shanahan, M. Kelly.
    Your over-35 week-by-week pregnancy guide : all the answers to all your questions about pregnancy, birth, and your developing baby / M. Kelly Shanahan.
      p. cm.
  Includes index.
  1. Pregnancy in middle age. 2. Pregnancy in middle age—Miscellanea.
  3. Childbirth in middle age—Miscellanea. I. Title: Your over-thirty-five week-by-week pregnancy guide. II. Title.

RG556.6 .S53 2000
618.2'4—dc21

00-050171

ISBN 0-7615-2698-6

10 9 8 7 6

First Edition

I DEDICATE THIS book to my mother, Barbara Dunn Shanahan. I used to call you an "old fart" because you had me when you were 35. I am older and wiser now, and am eternally grateful for everything you have done for me, Mom.

And to my husband, Jeff Turney. Without you, I wouldn't even have thought of having a child. Thank you for keeping me young at heart—and I promise I won't reveal your true age! Thank you for not only putting up with my normal contrariness, but for never complaining when I neglected my wifely duties writing this book.

And, mostly to my daughter, Hunter Katherine Shanahan Turney. Because of you, the M.D. after my name now stands for Mommy-Doctor. You are my little miracle, and I love you more than words can say. Thank you for being such a great kid and going to bed without a fuss so I could get to the computer. Thank you for not coloring, shredding, or otherwise destroying the research materials that cover every square inch of floor around my desk. Thank you for just being.

CONTENTS

PREFACE

IT WAS FATE when I was approached in early 2000 by Prima Publishing to write a book; in our family's annual holiday letter just a few weeks before, I had closed the letter with the comment that the only thing I hadn't yet done was to write a book! The proposed subject—a week-by-week guide to pregnancy after the age of 35—was fate as well. Not only am I a board-certified obstetrician-gynecologist, but the year before, at age 38, I gave birth to my first child. Been there, done that, write a book about it!

And writing this book was a lot like being pregnant. After the initial exhilaration ("Guess what, honey, they want me to write a book!"), there was the first-trimester anxiety ("What the heck am I going to write about? What did I get myself into?"). Then came the second-trimester honeymoon period, during which I was energized and could finish a chapter every day or two. But then came the third trimester ("I have to go sit in front of the computer again. I can't wait until this damn book is done!"). If you've already had a baby, you'll know what I mean, and if this is your first, the understanding will unfold, week by week.

Why did I want to write a book in the first place? Partly because I love to pass on what I know as an ob-gyn to other women. I could have limited my work to seeing my own patients four days a week, like most doctors do, but for the past few years I've been writing on the Internet, answering questions and writing articles for iVillage (allHealth.com), drugstore.com, and obgyn.net. I find great fulfill-ment in helping other women find answers to their questions and solutions to their problems. Writing a book, I felt, would be a logical extension of what I already love to do.

Why this book on pregnancy after 35? The time was ripe, for one thing. While in 1960 it was considered quite unusual that my mother had me, her first child, at age 35, today it is anything but uncommon. Today, more and more women are waiting until their mid- to late thirties—or even forties—to start a family. Some women who had their first children at a younger age complete their childbearing, either through choice or happenstance, after 35. There are special challenges and considerations—and, I believe, special joys—in being pregnant in our middle years. We have issues about chromosomal abnormalities that younger women don't. We are more likely to be troubled by complications like diabetes or high blood pressure. And, I think, we are more likely to be grateful to have the opportunity to be pregnant, and treasure each moment of it. When I started this book, my daughter was 14 months old. My experiences as an over-35-year-old pregnant woman were fresh in my mind. I wanted to pass on what I know as a doctor, to allay your fears and answer your questions. I also wanted to pass on what I know as a woman who had the same fears about being an older mom, the same questions about having genetic testing or not, the same joy in finally having a child. I went through infertility testing and treatments and two miscarriages before I was given the gift of being pregnant and having my daughter. I really have been there, done that.

This book is a resource for all women who find themselves "with child" at age 35 and beyond, whether they are first-time moms-to-be or veterans. It is arranged week-by-week; each chapter discusses what your baby is doing as well as what you are doing. Special considerations for each week are detailed, with emphasis on concerns of mid-life moms. I've included excerpts from the journal I kept when I was pregnant, because I thought the nine months of pregnancy were awesome, and I want to share that with you.

ACKNOWLEDGMENTS

THANKS GO TO Wendy Warner, M.D., in Yardley, Pennsylvania, for not only being a great friend, but for giving me such wonderful constructive criticism. To Cynthia Kolb, M.D., my associate, for reading the book, although I'm not sure if her effusive praise was because she really does think this is a great book, or because I make up the call schedule! To my friends and mentors at obgyn.net for answering obscure questions and providing feedback as well. To my editors at Prima: Libby Larson, who shepherded me through my first attempt at writing a book; and Lorna Eby, who approached me about writing a book in the first place. And mostly to my patients, who allowed me to quote them and to take their pictures on bad hair days!

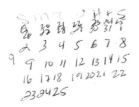

Your Over-35 Week-by-Week Pregnancy Guide

PREGNANCY PLANNING

You carry a Day Timer or Palm Pilot that has your week's activities scheduled to the minute. You budget for every expense, and you've never paid a bill late. You have an itinerary to account for every second of every day of your vacation. The birth of your child should be planned with the same care.

The Preconception Visit

One of the first things you should do once you've decided you'd like to have a baby is make an appointment with your ob-gyn and your general medical doctor, if you have one. This is especially important if you have any chronic medical conditions like asthma, diabetes, or high blood pressure. We over-35-year-olds are more likely to have chronic conditions than our younger sisters.

During a preconception visit, your doctor will ask you a lot of questions—ones you expect ("Do you have any medical problems?" "Have you had any surgery?" "Anybody in your family with cancer, diabetes, or high blood pressure?") as well as some you have probably never been asked before ("Have you had or been vaccinated for chicken pox?" "Anyone in your family with infertility or miscarriages?" "Do you work around chemicals?"). The answers to questions about whether you have ever been pregnant and what happened with each one can identify factors that may have contributed to miscarriages, preterm labor, or other poor outcomes in the past. You may be able to be screened for genetic diseases that can occur in people of your ethnic background or that run in your family. Table 1 lists some of the diseases for which carrier testing is available. Although you will be offered genetic testing because of your age (see week 10), if there is a family history of certain birth defects, mental retardation, or inherited conditions, you can undergo genetic counseling even before you try to get pregnant so that you may determine the risk of having an affected child.

TABLE 1
Carrier Testing Available

Condition	Who Should Be Tested
α-thalassemia	Southeast Asian or African ancestry
β-thalassemia	Mediterranean, Southeast Asian, Indian, Pakistani, or African ancestry
Cystic fibrosis	Positive family history
Fragile X syndrome	Family history of mental retardation
Sickle cell anemia	African, Caribbean, Mediterranean, Middle Eastern, Latin American, or Indian ancestry
Tay-Sachs	Eastern European Jewish (Ashkenazi), Cajun, or French Canadian ancestry

If you have a chronic medical condition like diabetes, high blood pressure, or seizures and are on medications, those medications may need to be adjusted. (This is discussed in detail in week 9.) Also, your medical condition should be as stable as possible before you get pregnant. This is especially true with diabetes; women who are diabetic are more likely to have babies with birth defects if their sugars are not well controlled at the time of conception.

Ideally, all immunizations should be brought up to date before getting pregnant. This would include the MMR (measles, mumps, and rubella), varicella (chicken pox), and hepatitis B vaccines.

Immunity to all of these can be assessed by a simple blood test during the preconception visit. If a vaccination is necessary, conception should be delayed 3 months. Also, if you are exposed to toxoplasmosis (cat owners), cytomegalovirus (workers in child care facilities, intensive care nurseries, or dialysis units), or tuberculosis (recent immigrant, live in crowded conditions), you can be tested to see if you are already immune to these diseases; if not, you will know to take special precautions to avoid contracting these infections during pregnancy.

Lifestyle issues are also extensively discussed during the preconception visit. It is best to get in shape and get to your ideal weight before getting pregnant. If your diet is primarily fast foods or prepared foods, now is the best time to learn new eating habits. If you smoke, you—and your partner if both of you smoke—should stop before you think about bringing a child into this world. Babies of parents who smoke are more likely to have asthma and other respiratory problems and to die from SIDS in their first year of life. You owe it to yourself and your baby to quit smoking before you conceive. The same goes for the use of illegal drugs or heavy drinking. And if you are a victim of domestic violence, don't think the abuse will stop once you get pregnant—talk to your doctor so you can get help before you bring a baby into an already volatile situation.

Your doctor will tell you about the importance of folic acid before conception and in the first few vital weeks of pregnancy. But just in case you get pregnant before that preconception visit, here's the scoop on folic acid: Folic acid helps lower the chance your baby will be born with a type of birth defect called *neural tube defects*. Sufficient levels must be present from the time fertilization happens, so all women who might get pregnant should get 0.4 mg (400 mcg) of folic acid daily. If you have had a child with spina bifida or another neural tube defect in the past, you should take 4 mg of folic acid beginning at least 1 month before getting pregnant and continuing for the first trimester. Folic acid is found in many foods such as spinach, whole grain breads, dried legumes, and citrus fruits, but for extra insurance, a supplement of 0.4 mg folic acid should be taken as well.

In addition to talking to your doctor, you should also talk to your health insurance agent and the benefits person at your workplace. You will need to find out if your current insurance plan covers pregnancy, and how much your deductible will be if pregnant. Also, explore your company's maternity leave policy. It is not too early to think about how much time you will want to take off after your baby is born, and what kind of disability benefits you will receive. If it is going to be difficult to pay all your bills without your full income, you can begin setting money aside now to offset your lost wages.

How to Get Pregnant

Okay, I know—or at least I hope—you know how to get pregnant! What I'm talking about is how to optimize your chances of getting pregnant. After all, you are older and it is a sad fact of nature that fertility declines with age. In any given month, a woman in her early twenties has a 25 percent chance of getting pregnant. In her late twenties to early thirties, that drops to 15 percent; we over-35-year-olds have only a 10 percent chance of getting pregnant in any given month, and that drops to 5 percent after age 40. While 95 percent of twenty-somethings will conceive within a year (taking an average of 4–5 months to do so), we over-35-year-olds have only a 65–70 percent chance, and it's likely to take us almost that whole year to be successful. Time is not on our side, ladies.

I'm not going to talk about infertility treatments here, as I could write an entire book on that subject, but if you have been trying to get pregnant for more than 6 months, and you are 35 or older, you should see your gynecologist to begin an infertility investigation. In general, about 40 percent of infertility is due to a male factor (low sperm count, poor sperm quality), 40 percent to a strictly female factor (not ovulating, blocked tubes), 10 percent to a little here and a little there, and the final 10 percent is unexplained. While 10–15 percent of all couples will have challenges getting pregnant, a third of women between 35 and 40, and a full half of women over 40 will be diagnosed with infertility.

In order to conceive, a sperm has to fertilize an egg. One or more eggs are released at *ovulation,* which usually happens about 14 days before you get your next period. The egg can only be fertilized within a 24-hour period after ovulation. Sperm, however, may survive in the reproductive tract for up to 5 days, leading to the concept of the "fertile window," this is the time frame in which an act of intercourse could potentially lead to pregnancy, and is 6 days total—the day of ovulation plus the 5 days before that. Your most fertile day is the day you ovulate, then the day before ovulation, and so forth. If you know when you are ovulating and make sure you have sex then, you will optimize your chances of getting pregnant. Having sex 2 days after you ovulate may be fun, but it's not going to get you a baby.

How can you tell when you ovulate? Ultrasound is the most reliable way, but face it, it is impractical and expensive, and should be reserved for women who are undergoing infertility treatments. Basal body temperature (BBT) charting is popular, but the rise in temperature does not happen until after ovulation occurs. BBTs can be useful to help you figure out when you usually ovulate, so you can make sure you are having sex around that time, but they cannot help you pinpoint ovulation in any given cycle. Cervical mucus can also be used as a clue; for a day or two right before and at ovulation, cervical mucus will become copious, clear, and stretchy, very reminiscent of egg whites. Table 3 outlines how to do and interpret BBTs, and the graph (table 2) shows BBTs and cervical mucus for an ovulatory cycle. Ovulation predictor test kits (OPKs) measure the surge in luteinizing hormone (LH; see week 2 for how LH stimulates ovulation), and a positive result precedes ovulation by 24–36 hours. An OPK can be used to make sure you have sex at your most fertile time, and can also be used to time special procedures like inseminations. I suggest OPKs rather than BBTs to my patients. I like the ability to use the test to time intercourse in a particular cycle. I like the ease of use (just urinate on a stick in the morning and wait for the result), and I myself could never do the BBTs— middle of the night phone calls, deliveries, and surgeries do not make for an accurate BBT!

If you are over 35 you'll need to put a little more effort into pregnancy planning. Take the time to see your doctor. Make the effort to get in shape and eat healthy. Think about how having a baby is going to change your life, and how you are going to adapt to those changes at home, at work, and at play. Discuss the risks of having a baby with a chromosomal abnormality with your partner, and begin to think about whether or not you will have genetic testing; it is a very difficult situation when you do not agree on this issue. Planning a pregnancy is exciting, like opening the pages of a new book—you don't know the ending, but you know you'll enjoy getting there.

TABLE 2

CYCLE DAY	1	2	3	4	5	6	7	8	9	10	11	12	13	14	15	16	17	18	19	20	21	22	23	24	25	26	27	28	29	30	31	32
DATE																																
TEMP															OVULATION																	
98.0																																
97.0																																
CERVICAL MUCUS											DRY/THICK	WET	WET, SLIPPERY	EGG WHITE	WET		DRY															
	PERIOD															3																

TABLE 3

Basal Body Temperature Charting

Doing the BBT

1. Buy a good quality digital thermometer or a glass fertility thermometer. The digital thermometer is faster. Special fertility thermometers only cover a small range of temperatures, so it is easier to read small differences than it would be with a regular thermometer.

2. Take your temperature first thing in the morning, before getting out of bed. If you forget and get up, or drink something, the temperature will be invalid.

3. Chart the result on graph paper. The horizontal axis is the day of your cycle (day 1 = the first day of your period) and the vertical axis is the temperature. There is an example of a BBT graph preceding.

4. Note things like a restless night, cold or flu, going to bed later than usual, and when you have sex on the chart.

Interpreting the BBT

1. Place a ruler horizontally along the 2 or 3 highest low temperatures. This is your coverline.

2. Look for a rise of at least $0.4°$ F ($0.2°$ C) from your coverline.

3. The temperature will remain elevated until you get your period. If you are pregnant, it will stay high.

4. The rise in temperature usually is abrupt and happens the day after ovulation.

Week 1 *(Start with first day of your last period)*

SUN _____ DATE 8/26

MON _____ DATE 8/20

⚡ TUE _____ DATE 8/21

WED _____ DATE 8/22

THUR _____ DATE 8/23

FRI _____ DATE 8/24

SAT _____ DATE 8/25

What Happened This Week?

_____

_____

_____

_____

How I Feel Physically and Emotionally

_____

_____

_____

_____

The Menstrual Cycle

TODAY, YOUR PERIOD begins. Be sure to jot this date down on your calendar: your doctor will use the first day of this *last menstrual period* (LMP) to determine your due date. Although you will not be pregnant for about another two weeks, today is the day your body starts the process that will culminate in your becoming a mother.

Also use this date to start the journal on page 8. You may want to use the journal to record important events and to note how you feel each week. If you're like me, you'll return to these pages over and over and over again—even after the baby is born.

How a Pregnancy Is Dated

Because most women do not know exactly when they ovulate and when they conceive, we use the first day of the last menstrual period to date pregnancies. The due date (EDC, or *estimated date of confinement,* a term left over from the days when women were put to bed for two weeks after giving birth) is 280 days—40 weeks—from the LMP. A quick way to determine your EDC is to count back

3 months from your LMP and add 7 days. For example, if the first day of your last menstrual period was April 10, back 3 months would be January, plus 7 days would be 17, for an EDC of January 17. This date has a margin of error of plus or minus 10 days, which is why it is called the "estimated" date.

The Menstrual Cycle

The first day of menstrual bleeding is designated cycle day 1. Menstrual bleeding happens because you did not get pregnant last month. *Progesterone* levels, which skyrocket after ovulation, drop precipitously if fertilization does not occur; this drop in progesterone leads to shedding of the uterine lining. Over the next few days, the *follicle* destined to ovulate begins to grow. Sometimes, there will be more than one dominant follicle recruited; this could result in fraternal twins. FSH, *follicle stimulating hormone,* is high at this point. FSH begins to stimulate production of estrogen around cycle day 5. Estrogen is necessary for growth of the soon-to-be-ovulated egg and also for growth of the uterine lining. FSH also begins to induce the formation of receptors for LH, *luteinizing hormone.* LH, as we will see in week 2, is vital for ovulation.

> ✎ DOCTOR'S MEMO
>
> Because I am an ob-gyn and because I am a woman, I use "doctor" throughout this book to refer to an obstetrician, a family practitioner, or a midwife, and her instead of the awkward he/she or him/her. I do not mean to imply that one type of practitioner—or gender of practitioner—is any better than the other.

Frequently Asked Questions

Q All I can think about is getting pregnant, but so far no luck. Friends have told me it's because I'm trying too hard. Is that possible?

A *While it is difficult to design a scientific approach to study it, the stress associated with trying too hard may impact fertility. Stress can lead to changes in hormone levels that are not conducive to conception. Because you are over 35, however, there are many, many other potential factors, so if you have been trying for over 6 months, see your doctor or a reproductive endocrinologist (fertility specialist) to have a few tests run.*

Q I like to take herbs and supplements. It it okay to continue taking these while I am trying to get pregnant?

A *There is a common misperception that if it is an herb it is safe and good; that just is not true—herbs are medicines, Mother Nature's pharmacy, if you will. Some herbs are safe for use in pregnancy, while others are extremely harmful, causing miscarriages or birth defects. You should never use any herb, over-the-counter, or prescription medication in pregnancy without clearing it with your own doctor, but here is a partial list of okay, maybe okay and never okay herbs in pregnancy:*

OKAY TO USE IN PREGNANCY
- Raspberry leaf
- Lemon balm
- Dandelion (but don't pick them from your yard if you use fertilizers or weed killers!)

MAY BE OKAY, UNDER THE SUPERVISION OF
A HEALTH CARE PROVIDER

- Echinacea
- Black cohosh (only in the last month of pregnancy to calm false labor)
- Ginger root

NEVER OKAY

- Ginseng
- Bloodroot
- Celery seed
- Chaparrel
- Comfrey
- Ma Huang (AKA ephedra)
- Fenugreek
- Feverfew
- Gingko
- Hops
- Hyssop
- Jimson weed
- Juniper
- Licorice (most licorice candies do not actually contain licorice, but only flavoring, which is okay)
- Nasturtium
- Pennyroyal
- Poppy
- Sage
- Sassafras
- Saw palmetto
- Senna
- Thyme (small amounts okay in cooking)
- Yucca

Q **I don't think I can make it through the day without coffee? Do I have to quit if I want to have a baby?**

A *You do not have to give up all of life's little indulgences in order to conceive and carry a healthy baby, but you do have to moderate. Research has shown that more than three servings of caffeine a day can increase the risk of miscarriage. Plus, caffeine is a diuretic, and can rob your body of vital fluids. My recommendation is to have only two caffeinated beverages a day. You can begin to wean yourself off the real stuff now, by mixing half regular and half decaf coffee. I went from two to three cups of coffee a day to two to three cups of decaf a week while I was trying to conceive—and I haven't gone back to the "leaded" version yet!*

Q **I am 42, remarried, and considering IVF (I had a tubal 8 years ago). My doctor wants me to have some blood work done on cycle day 3. Two questions: What is cycle day 3 and what is the blood test looking for?**

A *Since cycle day 1 is always the first day of menstrual bleeding, cycle day 3 is the third day of your period. Your doctor has probably ordered a FSH (follicle stimulating hormone) test. FSH helps stimulate egg development in preparation for ovulation. If the FSH is elevated on cycle day 3, then that suggests a poor egg reserve. In other words, you don't have a lot of good eggs left, and your chances of a successful outcome with IVF—or spontaneous conception—are low. In general, a cycle day 3 FSH> 15–20 mIU/ml (milli international units per milliliter) is a poor prognostic sign.*

Week 2

SUN   DATE 9\2

MON   DATE 9\3

TUE   DATE 8/28

WED   DATE 8/29

THUR   DATE 8/30

FRI   DATE 8/31

SAT   DATE 9\1

What Happened This Week?

How I Feel Physically and Emotionally

Ovulation and Fertilization

AT THE END of week 1, the menstrual flow has ended, and estrogen levels are rising, leading to growth of the dominant follicle (the egg destined to be ovulated); the uterine lining is beginning to thicken. This second week is chock-full of activity.

Ovulation

Thanks to estrogen, the uterine lining is growing from 0.5 mm to about 5 mm in thickness. The dominant follicle grows from 0.05 mm to 20 mm at the time of ovulation. Estrogen levels increase to 400 pg/ml (picogram/milliliter), 24–36 hours prior to ovulation, then begin to fall. The rapid increase in estrogen leads to a surge in luteinizing hormone (LH). Ovulation occurs twelve hours after peak LH levels are achieved. This LH surge is the basis of home ovulation predicting. Ovulation predictor kits (OPKs) test positive 24–36 hours prior to ovulation, allowing one to better time intercourse (see Pregnancy Planning).

Another interesting phenomenon that occurs during week 2 is an increase in *androgen* levels. Androgens are "male" hormones, but just as men have low levels of estrogen, women have low levels of testosterone. Non-dominant follicles, which started to grow earlier in the cycle, die off and produce androgens. This increase in androgen levels around the time of ovulation is thought to increase sexual desire in the woman, thus increasing the chances that she will have sex at a time that could lead to pregnancy! Mother Nature has all bases covered in her plan for us to continue reproducing.

The LH surge produces increases in progesterone. Progesterone acts on the follicle walls to increase distensibility (ability to expand, stretch, or fill with fluid). Fluid within the follicle rapidly accumulates. FSH, LH, and progesterone stimulate the activity of enzymes that break down the follicle wall. The follicle ruptures, the egg is released, and—voilà—ovulation has occurred!

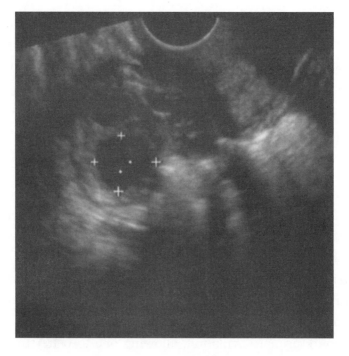

The large follicle (outlined by calipers) is the dominant follicle, about to be ovulated. A smaller follicle is also seen, just above. I just finished reading *Pinocchio* to that dominant follicle!

Fertilization

Once ovulation occurs, the egg (or eggs, if more than one was released) must come into contact with a sperm. While sperm can survive in your reproductive tract for up to 5 days, the egg is toast after 24 hours. This leads to the concept of the "fertile window," the time in which an act of intercourse could lead to a pregnancy. The fertile window encompasses the five days before ovulation and the day of ovulation; the day on which sex is most likely to lead to pregnancy is the day of ovulation, followed by the day before ovulation, and so on.

When a man ejaculates, he deposits between 200 and 300 *million* sperm into the woman's vagina. Of those millions and millions of sperm, only about 200 get near the egg. During the journey from vagina, through the cervix and uterus, and into the tubes, the sperm undergo a process called *capacitation,* which gives sperm the ability to attach to and penetrate the egg. Once one sperm attaches to the egg, a reaction occurs that prevents other sperm from gaining entry. The genetic material from the victorious sperm and the egg join and fuse—and your baby is begun!

At the time of fertilization, the 23 *chromosomes* from Dad and the 23 chromosomes from Mom are joined into 23 pairs of chromosomes, one from each parent. These chromosomes determine hair and eye color, height, body type, and everything else about your baby. The chromosomes are matched, with the exception of the sex chromosomes, X and Y. Females have two X chromosomes and males have one X and one Y. The egg always supplies an X, but the sperm can supply an X or a Y; if a Y-bearing sperm fertilizes the egg (for an XY combination), the result will be a boy, but if the sperm carries an X (for an XX), you'll have a girl. If Dad complains about what he gets, remind him that he determines the gender of his children!

Frequently Asked Questions

Q I have a friend with a blue-eyed daughter, but my friend and her husband have brown eyes—how can that be?

A *This is a good example of recessive and dominant genes—and not a sign your friend was friendly with the milkman! We have two copies of each gene (with the exception of males, who have one X chromosome from mom and one Y chromosome from dad); some genes are dominant, meaning only one copy is required to express that gene's trait, while others are recessive—both copies are needed for that trait to be expressed. The gene for brown eyes is dominant, while blue (and green) are recessive. Your friend and her husband each have one brown and one blue gene (but remember, brown is dominant, hence they each have brown eyes). They each gave a blue gene to their daughter—two copies of blue equals blue eyes. Similarly, brown or black hair is dominant, while blonde or red is recessive.*

Q I know I am paranoid, but what if I have some odd genetic problem, but don't know about it?

A *If you have an isolated genetic defect, and you are fine, it is unlikely that you will meet up with a man with the same defect and you both pass the defect on to your child, and have your child be adversely affected by it.*

Cystic fibrosis is one of the more common genetic defects in Caucasians, with 1:20 carrying the gene; this translates into a 1:400 chance of a baby having cystic fibrosis. Now, if there are birth defects in the family, even in distant relatives, then genetic counseling may be helpful. We do not have the technology—or the financial resources— to screen every single person for every single genetic problem.

Q I'm 36 and trying to have my first baby. My best friend says she can always tell when she is ovulating because she has pain off to one side in her pelvic area. I've never felt this. Does this mean I'm not ovulating?

A *Your friend is having mittleschmertz, German for "middle pain." This short lived, usually sharp pain lasts for several hours to a day midcycle, around ovulation. Some women feel it, but many do not. You can be ovulating every month and never have a twinge. You can always do an ovulation predictor test to see if you are ovulating, and, remember, if you have been trying for more than 6 months, see your doctor for an evaluation.*

Week 3

SUN   DATE 9/9

MON   DATE 9/10

TUE   DATE 9/4

WED   DATE 9/5

THUR   DATE 9/6

FRI   DATE 9/7

SAT   DATE 9/8

What Happened This Week?

How I Feel Physically and Emotionally

20

Implantation

FERTILIZATION IS THE first step on the long journey that will end in the delivery room. From now on, for each week I will explain what your baby is doing, what you are doing, and what the special considerations are for that week.

What Baby Is Doing

Right now, your baby certainly does not look like a baby. Once fertilization occurs and the genetic material from sperm (Dad) and egg (Mom) joins together, the 1 cell formed begins to divide. Over the course of the next 3 days, this cell, as it travels down the fallopian tube toward the uterus, will slowly divide into two, then four, then eight cells, called *blastomeres*. A solid ball of 12–16 cells, called a *morula*, enters the uterine cavity about 3 days after fertilization. Fluid begins to accumulate between the blastomeres, forming a *blastocyst*, with a bunch of cells at one end that will eventually be your baby and a rim of cells (*trophoblasts*) all around. During this stage, your baby is called a *zygote*.

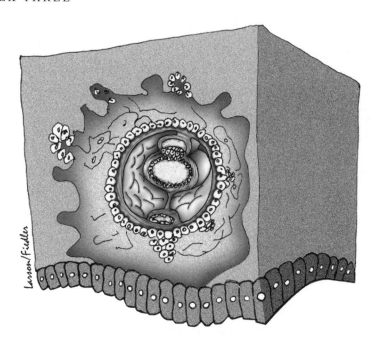

This drawing illustrates a blastocyte a few days after implantation has occurred. The embryonic disc lies between the smaller amniotic cavity on the top and the larger primary yolk sac on the bottom.

During the next 72 hours, the zygote floats around in the uterine cavity. Six or 7 days after fertilization, at the end of week 3, it implants into the thick, lush uterine lining (see next section for what your body has been doing to prepare for this). At this point, your baby is composed of between 107 and 256 cells and measures 0.15 mm—about the size of a period on this page! Implantation usually occurs in the upper, back wall of the uterus; implantation in the lower portion of the uterus may result in a *placenta previa* (see week 25). The trophoblast cells burrow between the uterine lining cells, until the zygote is completely covered by the uterine lining.

The trophoblasts (and their descendants, the fetal membranes and placenta) are the only cells that come into direct contact with maternal tissue and blood. One of the great mysteries of human reproduction is why Mom's body does not reject a baby. After all, the developing baby is a mix of your genes and those of your partner; it is genetically different from you, and therefore foreign. Our bodies are very good at rejecting foreign invaders—think of our response to infection, or the need for people who have received transplanted organs to take powerful drugs to avoid rejection of the organ. Why doesn't our body reject this tiny bundle of cells invading the uterine lining? Doctors and scientists think there is something special about the trophoblasts that "trick" Mom's body into thinking the developing baby is not foreign tissue. I like to think of it as one of many miracles associated with having a child.

What You Are Doing

While the egg and sperm were getting to know one another, your body was keeping pretty busy, too. Under the influence of estrogen, glands within your uterine lining (*endometrium*, in medical terms) are growing and becoming more branched and tortuous. At the time of implantation, the uterine lining has increased to 10–14 mm in thickness. Active secretion from the glands produces a fluid in which the zygote (scheduled to arrive in the uterus the middle of this third week) will be bathed until it implants in the uterine lining at the end of this week. Many of these secretions are necessary for successful implantation.

Your ovary has been busy, too. The site of ovulation, now called the *corpus luteum*, is producing great quantities of progesterone. Progesterone is required to support the pregnancy until the placenta begins to secrete sufficient amounts, around week 10. If the corpus luteum is disrupted, a miscarriage will occur unless supplemental progesterone is given.

All of these things happening in your body occur without any conscious input from you. You will not feel any different than normal at this point—breast tenderness, nausea, showing, and glowing are all to come.

Special Considerations

Shortly after implantation, some women will experience spotting. As your baby burrows into the uterine lining, small blood vessels may be disrupted. This bleeding is usually very light and lasts only a day or so. It is sometimes red and sometimes brownish. Because it occurs close to the time of an expected period, many women mistake this spotting for a period and do not realize until several weeks later that they are pregnant.

Frequently Asked Questions

Q I am trying to conceive and I may have ovulated about a week ago. Tonight is our tenth anniversary. Is it okay for me to have some champagne?

A *Even if you did conceive last week, the baby probably has not implanted yet, so there is no connection between you and the baby. Any alcohol you drink, therefore, will not be passed on. It is fine to enjoy your anniversary dinner; if you are pregnant, anniversary number 11 will be spent burping baby and changing diapers!*

Q I had a little spotting today, but my period is not due for a few more days. I really want to be pregnant. Can I do a pregnancy test yet?

A *A very sensitive blood pregnancy test may be positive the day after implantation, but home tests will not be. If you do not have a full-blown period within a few days of when it was due, spotting may be from implantation and you should do a home pregnancy test. While the waiting game is difficult, if you think of it as an exercise in the patience you will need once you have a child, it is more tolerable!*

Q I did a home pregnancy test because I just felt pregnant. My last period started only 15 days ago, but the test was positive. I thought I had to miss a period before a pregnancy test would be positive?

A *You do not have to miss a period before a sensitive pregnancy test will register the result; however, the implantation must have occurred before HCG can be detected. Implantation occurs around 6 days after fertilization, so unless you ovulated unusually early this cycle, implantation would not have occurred yet.*

What is more likely is that your last period wasn't really a period at all, but rather implantation bleeding and you conceived last month! Make an appointment with your doctor for an exam, a blood HCG level, and perhaps an ultrasound to determine exactly how far along you are.

Week 4

SUN   DATE 9/16

MON   DATE 9/17

✗ TUE   DATE 9/11

WED   DATE 9/12

THUR   DATE 9/13

FRI   DATE 9/14

SAT   DATE 9/15

What Happened This Week?

_____

_____

_____

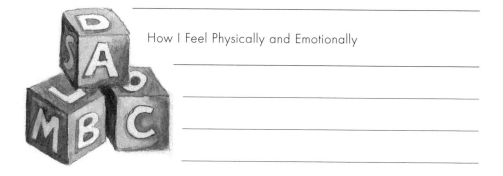

How I Feel Physically and Emotionally

_____

_____

_____

_____

Where's My Period?

At the end of this week, you may be wondering where the heck your period is and beginning to suspect you are pregnant. Blood pregnancy tests will be positive early in the week, and home urine tests generally will reveal the good news the first day of a missed period.

What Baby Is Doing

Your baby has been producing HCG (*human chorionic gonadotropin*), the pregnancy hormone, since 2 to 3 days after fertilization. Now that implantation has occurred, a connection between your blood and the trophoblasts is being established. Using very sensitive blood tests, HCG can be detected in your blood the day after implantation. This hormone is extremely important; it signals your body that you are pregnant (see next section for what your body does in response to HCG).

During this week your baby zygote becomes an *embryo*, as it will be called until the tenth week. The bunch of cells at one end of the blastocyst (discussed in week 3) begins to form distinct layers and is now called the *embryonic disc*. A small cavity, the precursor to the *amniotic cavity*, forms as well. On the opposite side of the embryonic disc from the amniotic cavity, the *yolk sac* begins to form. The yolk sac is important in the transfer of nutrients to the developing embryo, and next week will begin supplying blood cells.

By the end of this week, the deepest layer of trophoblasts have formed tiny finger-like projections and are now called *chorionic villi*. Some of your blood vessels are invaded by these cells, establishing the maternal-fetal connections that will supply the developing baby with nutrients and oxygen and will take away wastes until delivery.

At the end of this week, your baby is 0.4–1.0 mm in length— about the size of a grain of sand.

What You Are Doing

HCG from the baby signals the corpus luteum to continue to produce progesterone; without this signal, the corpus luteum would degenerate, progesterone levels would fall, and a period would begin. High levels of progesterone and estrogen stimulate continued growth of the uterine lining and promote the *decidual reaction*. The decidual changes in the uterine lining help ensure the success of implantation and supply nourishment to the baby until the placental circulation is established. By the end of this week, the site of implantation is covered by a layer of decidual cells.

From My Journal
"3/29/98. + UHCG [urine pregnancy test] yesterday!!!! It's funny, I don't feel pregnant—breasts aren't particularly full and tender like they have been before [I had 2 miscarriages before my daughter]. I hope the little spirit(s) have taken hold. . . ."

Soon after implantation occurs, early in this fourth week, tiny blood vessels in the uterine lining are invaded by the trophoblasts.

This establishes a connection between you and the developing baby. HCG produced by the baby can now enter your circulatory system and be detected by blood and, a few days later, urine tests.

At this point, you may feel as if you are about to get a period— you may have a sensation of pelvic fullness or heaviness and your breasts may tingle a bit. Your uterus is the same size as it was pre-pregnancy and examination alone is not adequate to confirm pregnancy.

Special Considerations

Now that there is a physical connection between you and the baby (some women feel an emotional connection from the moment of conception), your actions can affect the baby. Smoking, drinking alcohol, using drugs, or exposure to chemicals can have long-term consequences for this rapidly dividing group of cells in you. (This is discussed extensively in week 9.)

This connection also allows you to find out you are pregnant. As explained earlier, once endometrial blood vessels are invaded by the trophoblasts, HCG secreted by the baby enters your circulation. Sensitive blood tests can detect this HCG as early as the day after implantation, or right at the beginning of

✎ DOCTOR'S MEMO

Watching urine move across the test stick of a home pregnancy test is an exciting moment for many women. One of my patients wrapped the test up, placed it on the kitchen table where her husband sat and watched his expressions change from bewilderment ("It's not my birthday"), to confusion ("What the heck is this thing?") to utter joy when he figured out what it meant ("I'm gonna be a dad!").

week 4. Unless you have been undergoing infertility treatments, it is unlikely you will have a blood test done so soon. By the end of this week, right around the time you should be getting a period, however, you may suspect you are pregnant and wish to do a test. By the day you expect your period, over-the-counter home pregnancy tests can detect HCG that is passed into your urine. One brand, First Response, received FDA approval in early 2000 to market a home test that can detect HCG three days before a period is due! Home tests are much less expensive than blood tests, and are 99 percent accurate. False negatives (indicating you are not pregnant when you really are) are much more common than false positives. If you do a test and get a negative result, retest a few days later. Sometimes we ovulate—and therefore conceive—a few days later than we think, so the entire timetable, including HCG's appearance in your system, is delayed. Because home tests are so accurate, it is not necessary under most circumstances to have a positive test repeated in your doctor's office.

Frequently Asked Questions

Unless you have undergone infertility treatments, you will probably not see your doctor yet. If you have had a prior *ectopic pregnancy* or multiple miscarriages, call your doctor now. Blood tests for HCG levels may be done to determine whether this pregnancy is in the proper place. With an ectopic pregnancy, HCG levels will not rise properly. (This is discussed in detail in week 8.) If you have had miscarriages or been diagnosed with a *luteal phase defect,* your doctor may wish to test progesterone levels as well; if low, progesterone supplements may help prevent another miscarriage. (See week 8 for more information on ectopic pregnancy and miscarriage.)

Q I did a home pregnancy test, but the line is very faint. What does this mean?

A *It means you are pregnant. Unlike ovulation predictor testing (see Pregnancy Planning), the darkness of the line on a home pregnancy test does not factor into the interpretation of positive versus negative; any second line is considered positive. The line may be fainter because you are very early, or because your urine was more dilute, lowering the concentration of HCG in the sample. The darkness of the line tells nothing about the health of the baby or whether you will miscarry or have a tubal pregnancy. All it does is let you know you need to call your doctor for a prenatal appointment!*

Q I know I'm pregnant (woman's intuition, or something), but the pregnancy test is negative and my period is three days late.

A *I am a firm believer in woman's intuition. Some women just do not produce HCG that can be detected on home tests. Sometimes you ovulate later than you think and there may not be any HCG in your system yet. Retest in a few days, when levels may be higher. (Retest using your first morning urine, because it is more concentrated and lower levels of HCG may be detected.) If the test is still negative, see your doctor for a blood test and exam. The blood tests are much more sensitive than the urine tests.*

Q I did a pregnancy test this morning and it was positive! Father's Day is in two weeks and I'd love to wrap the stick up and give it to my husband with a card, to let him know we're going to have a baby. Assuming I can keep a secret for two weeks, will the test still register positive?

A *That is a great way to tell Dad-to-be the good news! And, yes, the positive result will still show. In theory, a second line will remain indefinitely. I have a couple of patients who have kept the stick for the baby's keepsake box, but I must admit I don't know if they've looked at it since the baby was born.*

Week 5

SUN   DATE   9/23

MON   DATE   9/24

TUE   DATE 9/18

WED   DATE 9/19

THUR   DATE 9/20

FRI   DATE 9/21

SAT   DATE   9/22

What Happened This Week?

How I Feel Physically and Emotionally

Why Am I So Tired??

DURING THIS WEEK, you may begin to feel pregnant. You may notice a surprising (to first-time moms) sense of fatigue, and your breasts may be very sensitive. Your baby is changing every day, and equally significant changes have already begun in your body.

What Baby Is Doing

Last week, the baby consisted of two layers; this week a third layer forms. The *ectoderm* will become skin, hair, the nervous system, the lenses of the eyes, and tooth enamel; the *endoderm* will develop into the lungs and digestive system; and the *mesoderm* becomes the skeleton, muscles, urinary system, reproductive system, and circulatory system. A groove, called the *neural groove*, is forming down the baby's back. The neural groove will begin to fold over, forming the *neural tube*. The neural tube eventually becomes the spinal cord, brain, and nervous system. If this process is disturbed, abnormalities of the brain and spinal cord (*neural tube defects*) such as spina bifida or anencephaly may result (see week 15).

By the end of this week, several *somites*, looking like stacked-up blocks, form on either side of the neural tube; these somites are the precursors to muscle and bone. The cardiovascular system is beginning to form as well. First, small blood vessels begin to form from mesodermal cells in the baby as well as in the yolk sac and chorionic villi. A primitive heart tube develops in the chest area and connects with these blood vessels. Blood cells develop from the lining of the yolk sac and are circulated through the baby when the tubular heart begins to beat at the end of this week.

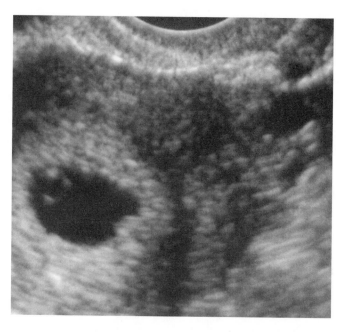

"The yolk sac is the circle on the left. The baby—a "fetal pole" at this stage—is not visible. Black is the amniotic fluid. Other structures, like the wall of the yolk sac, are shades of gray. The brighter gray ring around the black amniotic sac reflects the decidual reaction caused by our friend progesterone."

The entire *gestational* sac, the embryo and its surrounding fluid and membranes, is about 1 cm in diameter. Your baby measures about 1.5 mm—about the size of the lowercase 'o' on this page.

What You Are Doing

Your uterus has not grown yet, although it may feel a bit softer on a pelvic exam. You have not gained any weight (or at least you shouldn't have!) yet either. Significant changes are occurring, however, even if you cannot see them.

Progesterone levels continue to increase. In addition to its importance in sustaining the early pregnancy, progesterone has profound impacts on you. It is almost sedative in nature, contributing to the fatigue that affects almost all pregnant women (see Special Considerations). It also slows down the intestinal tract and may contribute to constipation and bloating. If you have had a baby before, you may feel that you are much larger than the first time; the progesterone bloat, combined with previously stretched out abdominal muscles, may lead to tight pants this soon!

Progesterone also stimulates growth of the milk-producing glands in the breast, leading to a sensation of fullness and tingling, even this early. Blood volume has already begun to increase, but red cell mass has not; this eventually leads to the anemia that is so common in pregnancy. The composition of blood plasma begins to change dramatically around the fifth week as well, which contributes to fluid retention.

Special Considerations

It is amazing to most women how utterly exhausted they can be so early in pregnancy. The baby is not much bigger than a speck, but already you want to sleep all the time. Because you are over 35, you might be tempted to blame your age. Don't: 25-year-olds are tired, too. Progesterone, with its sedative effects, does not discriminate based on age. One difference between younger moms-to-be and older ones, however, is that we over-35-year-olds just may have more on our plates in the first place. And if you already have small children, well, of course you are going to be exhausted!

✎ DOCTOR'S NOTES

When I was 25, I was in med school, and while it was rigorous, all I did was go to class and study. When I was 38 and pregnant with my daughter, in addition to my full-time ob-gyn practice, I was chairperson of my hospital's ob-gyn department; in charge of a significant chunk of a charity fund-raiser scheduled for 3 weeks before my due date; writing weekly columns and doing chats for iVillage.com and obgyn.net; and on the board of the local Soroptimist chapter!

Fatigue is also a signal from your body to take care of yourself so that you can take care of this baby developing inside you. Take naps when you can. Delegate household chores to your significant other. You didn't get pregnant by yourself, you don't eat all the food or generate all the laundry—he can't carry the baby for you, but he sure can vacuum and go to the grocery store. Learn how to say "No" when asked to take on additional responsibilities both on and off the job (here is an example of do what I say, not what I do!).

In addition to a desire to sleep the entire day and night, you may start to notice that your breasts are very tender. They may be a bit larger already, too. Many dads-to-be are thrilled at your new curves, until they hear, "Don't even think about touching them—and don't even look at them, they hurt so much!" Wearing a supportive bra (sports bras work well), even to bed, can help with this discomfort.

Frequently Asked Questions

If you do not have a doctor or midwife already, now is the time to find one! Obstetricians are doctors who have undergone a 4-year residency program after medical school, specializing in all aspects of female reproductive health, including the management of pregnancies and delivery by all methods. Family practitioners in some areas may also deliver babies. Family practitioners do a 3-year residency, with several months devoted to obstetrics and gynecology; most family practitioners do not follow high-risk pregnancies or do cesarean sections, but will call upon an obstetrician in these cases. Certified nurse-midwives are nurses who have done additional training beyond nursing school in order to care for and deliver low-risk pregnancies; they often have a more "touchy-feely" approach than doctors. Midwives work under the supervision of an obstetrician, whom they will call if there are any complications. You will be seeing your doctor or midwife from now until delivery, so it is important you are comfortable, not only with her qualifications, but also with her personality and style.

If you are looking for a doctor or midwife, or if you have only seen your doctor for gynecological care, here are some questions you might want to ask:

Q Where do you deliver babies?

A *This may seem like a no-brainer in a small community, but in a larger city, your doc may have privileges at several hospitals.*

Q Do you accept my insurance?

A *Ask the front office staff this question. If your doc is anything like me, she won't know!*

Q Who will do my delivery if you are not available? Will I meet this person during the course of my prenatal care?

A *Many doctors—and midwives—practice as part of a group, so you will meet all members, and the one who happens to be on call when you go into labor will be the one having the privilege of doing your delivery. If your doc is not part of a group, she will make arrangements for another person to cover, but you may not be able to meet that person ahead of time.*

Week 6

SUN   DATE 9/30

MON   DATE 10/1

TUE   DATE 9/25

WED   DATE 9/26

THUR   DATE 9/22

FRI   DATE 9/28

SAT   DATE 9/29

What Happened This Week?

_____

_____

_____

_____

How I Feel Physically and Emotionally

_____

_____

_____

_____

First Doctor's Visit

M ANY WOMEN WILL see their doctors for the first time this week. Some practices do not schedule visits until about the tenth week. Others may have you come in, speak with a nurse, and have lab work done, but not have you see the doctor until a few weeks later.

What Baby Is Doing

This week marks the beginning of *organogenesis*, the time in which all the major internal and external structures are formed; this period lasts until week 10, although growth and increasing function continue even after birth. During this stage, exposure to drugs, chemicals, or infections may cause birth defects (see week 9).

During this sixth week (fourth week after conception), your baby begins to fold and takes on a characteristic C-shape. A large prominence on the inner portion of the C (the baby's "front") marks the location of the by-now functional heart. In the middle of this week, tiny arm buds form, followed by leg buds. Pits on the side of the head, which will become the inner ear, are visible, as are thick-

From My Journal

"4/17/98. We saw your heartbeat today!! That little flicker is the most beautiful sight. I hope and pray every day that you have taken root well, and will continue to grow strong. We really want you to stay with us and be our child. . . . "

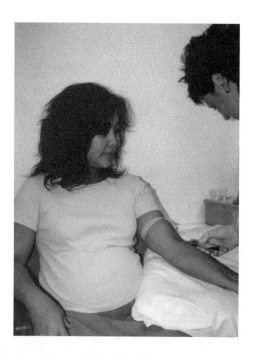

Drucilla, age 35, has blood for one of her pre-natal lab tests drawn.

enings that are the forerunners of the lenses of the eyes. The head end of the neural tube closes by the end of this week.

Your baby has grown to 4 mm long, the size of a grain of rice. The heart is beating and can be seen on trans-vaginal ultrasound most of the time.

What You Are Doing

At this point, your uterus has enlarged enough that your doctor should be able to tell you are pregnant by a pelvic exam; the normally navel orange–sized uterus is the size of a small grapefruit now. If you are overweight, however, this may still be difficult to feel. Your breasts are fuller, although if you have had a baby before, this may not be noticeable; first-time moms may have already had to go up a bra size. I went from an A-cup to a D-cup when I was pregnant with my daughter and had cleavage for the first (and only) time in my life!

You may have gained a pound or two, but if you have not, don't worry. I recommend minimal weight gain in the first trimester. Some women, plagued by morning sickness, may have actually lost weight. (We'll talk about morning sickness extensively in week 7.) Most first-time moms can still fit into their jeans, but if you have had a baby before, you may be losing your waistline already; the combination of bloating caused by high progesterone levels and previously stretched-out abdominal muscles cause many a second-time mom to resort to leggings and big shirts even this early.

Special Considerations

You will probably see your doctor for your first prenatal visit this week. I encourage you to bring your partner with you for this visit; in addition to the fact that it took "two to tango" in the first place, it is important for your doctor to get information about his family history as well. If you used donor sperm for any reason (choice of single parenthood, lesbian relationship, low or no sperm count on your husband's part), bring any information the sperm bank provided regarding the donor's background.

First, you will be asked numerous questions about your medical, gynecological, surgical, social, and family history (see table 6.1). It is important to answer these questions as completely and honestly as possible, as the answers may place you in a higher or lower risk category (all of us over-35-year-olds are in a slightly higher risk group anyway, merely because of our age!).

Next, you will have a complete physical, unless you have had one very, very recently. Your doctor will examine you head to toe, with emphasis, of course, on the pelvic exam. A pap smear will be done, as well as tests for infections such as gonorrhea and chlamydia. The size of your uterus will be assessed by a *bimanual exam*, the typical pelvic exam in which your doctor will place two fingers in your vagina and the other hand on your lower abdomen to feel how big your uterus is and to get an idea of how far along you are.

Blood work is usually drawn at this first visit as well. A routine

TABLE 6.1

Typical Prenatal Questionnaire

Have you or anyone in your family (blood relatives) had

1. Birth defects?
2. Genetic diseases?
3. Twins or other multiple births?
4. Diabetes?
5. High blood pressure?
6. Lung disease?
7. Kidney disease?
8. Neurologic disease?
9. Psychiatric disorders?
10. Endocrine or metabolic diseases?
11. Blood disorders?

Do you now, or have you

1. Experienced infertility?
2. Had venereal disease or abnormal pap smear?
3. Had previous pregnancies? What was the outcome of each?
4. Smoked cigarettes?
5. Drunk alcohol?
6. Used recreational drugs?
7. Had allergy to medications?
8. Had operations or accidents?
9. Had previous hospitalizations?
10. Had blood transfusions, tattoos or sex with an IV drug user?
11. Own pets, especially cats?
12. Experienced exposure to chemicals at work or home?

prenatal panel consists of blood type, including Rh factor; syphilis; rubella (German measles); hepatitis B surface antigen; blood count; and HIV (standard in most practices). If there is a personal or family history of diabetes, a blood sugar test may be done as well. Although it is far from standard as I write this (mid-2000), testing for an underactive thyroid may become part of the panel, too; recent studies have shown that undiagnosed or undertreated hypothyroidism in moms may contribute to lower IQs in babies. (See week 13 for interpretation of all these tests.)

✎ DOCTOR'S NOTES

One hint for easier prenatal visits: Don't wear jumpsuits or overalls. Your doctor will need to get to your belly to measure your uterus and listen to your baby, so two-piece outfits are much easier! Not to mention at this point you are probably urinating a lot, and overalls or jumpsuits are not the most bathroom-friendly articles of clothing.

Frequently Asked Questions

Here are some typical questions people ask during the first visit—because forgetfulness is common throughout pregnancy, jot down questions as you think of them, and then try to remember to bring the paper with you each visit!

Q **I am not tired, my breasts don't hurt, and I'm not sick at all. Does this mean something is wrong?**

A *No, it just means you are lucky! And don't start bragging to all your friends yet—you may start throwing up next week! While the symptoms you mention are common in pregnancy, some women do not get any of them. These very fortunate few sail through their pregnancies with nary an upset stomach, varicose vein, or hair out of place and still deliver wonderfully healthy babies.*

Q I am terrified my husband will find out I had an abortion before we were married. Do I have to tell my doctor?

A *It is important to tell your doctor about previous pregnancies, sexually transmitted diseases, drug, alcohol, and tobacco use because these things can affect this pregnancy and this baby. While one first-trimester abortion will have no adverse effects on this pregnancy, multiple prior abortions or a second-trimester abortion may increase your risk of complications such as an incompetent cervix; your doctor will not know to look for potential problems unless you are honest with her. You could tell her in private, and ask that this information be kept confidential.*

Q I break out in a cold sweat at the thought of having a pelvic exam. Will I have one every visit?

A *Oh, my, no—that would be awful! This first visit does require a pelvic exam and pap smear, but most of your visits will not require you to take off anything more than your shoes (I haven't seen a woman yet not remove shoes, purse, sweater and anything else she can before getting on the scale!). After the complete physical this visit, most of your prenatal visits will entail providing a urine sample, having your weight and blood pressure recorded, listening to the baby's heartbeat (after 8–10 weeks), and making sure your uterus measures what it should for that point in the pregnancy (actual measuring with a tape measure usually after 20 weeks; between 12 and 20 weeks your doctor will just feel where it is in relationship to your pubic bone and belly button).*

Q I own my own business and it is so hard for me to take the time for these prenatal visits. If I feel okay, why do I have to see the doctor anyway?

A *There are multiple reasons to make the time to see your doctor regularly throughout your pregnancy. One is that many of the warning signs for pregnancy complications are subtle and you may not notice them. Studies have shown that women who have regular prenatal care beginning early in pregnancy are less likely to experience preterm labor or low birth weight babies. Diabetes may go undiscovered unless you have the glucola test (discussed in Week 28) or you spill excess sugar in your urine. If your blood pressure is not checked regularly, it could cause harm to your baby if not treated appropriately. Another reason to have regular visits is to establish a relationship with your doctor(s) and to have opportunities to discuss questions you may have about the progress of your pregnancy, as well as what to expect in the delivery room.*

Week 7

SUN   DATE 10/7

travel back to scc

MON   DATE 10/8

TUE   DATE 10/2

WED   DATE 10/3

THUR   DATE 10/4

travel to NYC

FRI   DATE 10/5

SAT   DATE 10/6

What Happened This Week?

light cramping in my back

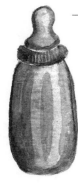

How I Feel Physically and Emotionally

Greg came home Wednesday smelling of
garlic - couldn't stand to be around him -
1st real big emotional melt down - feeling
over welmed -
Smells really starting to bother me

Morning (and Noon and Night) Sickness

IF YOU ARE in the majority of pregnant women, expect the queasies to hit in full force this week. If you are in the lucky minority who do not experience morning sickness, take my advice and don't mention that to any other pregnant women in your doctor's waiting room!

What Baby Is Doing

All the organ systems that began developing last week are continuing to grow and to differentiate. The head grows much more than the rest of the body, due to rapid development of the brain. The head curves over and touches the chest, so that your baby looks like a tiny little shrimp.

On the baby's head, a *lens placode* (the precursor to the lens of the eye) is now visible. Nasal pits and a primitive mouth form as well. In the respiratory system, the tiny lung bud at the end of the trachea branches again into two bronchial buds that will become the right and left main stem bronchi. The heart, a mere tube just last week, begins to divide into chambers and arteries, and veins are in place to all the other developing organs. Blood cells are still produced in the yolk sac at this point.

In the abdomen, the intestines and digestive system are well on their way. One side of the stomach grows more than the other, so it already has the normal adult hockey stick shape. The duodenum, the portion of small bowel that connects with the stomach, is solid at this point, rather than a hollow tube. The liver, gallbladder, and spleen all form this week as well, although they do not yet function. Two mesonephric ridges, forerunners of the kidneys, develop on either side of the baby's back.

Your baby is a whopping 8mm long now, about the size and shape of a Cheerio cut in half.

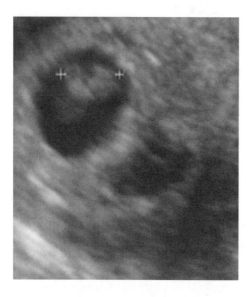

"This tiny baby, outlined by the calipers, already has a heartbeat!"

What You Are Doing

At this point, you may notice some subtle changes in your body, particularly in your breasts. They will be fuller, and the areola, the pigmented area around the nipples, may be darker and bigger around. Blood vessels may be more prominent. Your belly will not be noticeably bigger for several more weeks, although your uterus continues to grow. You should not be gaining any significant amounts of weight yet, and may be losing small amounts due to nausea and an increased metabolic rate.

Special Considerations

Morning sickness is one of the most inaccurate terms ever coined; it doesn't just happen in the morning, it can occur at any time, in any place, with any trigger. More than 50 percent of all pregnant women experience nausea to one degree or another. For most, it is an annoying rite of passage on the way to becoming a mother. For others, it is full-fledged vomiting that interferes with normal daily functioning and may require hospitalization. Severe morning sickness, called *hyperemesis gravidarum*, affects 2 percent of pregnancies.

Morning sickness occurs because of high levels of HCG. When HCG levels begin to decline, around 12–14 weeks, so does morning sickness. A rare woman will be queasy throughout her entire pregnancy, however. High estrogen levels also contribute to morning sickness. This is the basis for the old wives' tale that we are more sick when pregnant with girls than with boys, although in my practice, I think boys cause as much nausea as girls.

There are as many remedies for morning sickness as there have been women hunched over toilet bowls (see table 7.1). Some have been handed down through the

> ## ✎ DOCTOR'S NOTES
>
> When I was pregnant with my daughter, I threw up every day from 7 to 13 weeks. It didn't matter whether I ate or not; 30 minutes after I got up, I threw up, and that was it for the day. I just got up earlier to compensate for the extra time! I was so thankful to be pregnant at all, to not have miscarried already, that the morning sickness didn't bother me— at least not mentally. Physically, vomiting is vomiting, no matter how happy you are to be doing it.

TABLE 7.1

Helpful Hints for Morning Sickness

1. Eat two or three crackers or pretzels when you first wake up. Stay in bed for 15–20 minutes afterward.

2. Drink ginger or peppermint tea immediately upon awakening (have your mate brew it and bring it to you).

3. Do not eat solid food and drink liquids at the same time. Wait 30 minutes after eating to drink, or vice versa.

4. Eat frequent, small meals. Combinations of carbohydrates and protein work best for most women.

5. Ginger tea or ginger root capsules can be very effective for morning sickness. Do not take ginger root capsules if you have had a miscarriage before; ginger tea is okay, however.

6. Sniff a cut lemon or a rubbing alcohol wipe. It may sound silly, but sniffing an alcohol wipe got me through many a surgery during my pregnancy!

7. Take vitamin B6, 25 mg, up to three times a day. This has been found to be effective in several well-designed scientific studies.

8. There is a spot between the two tendons on the underside of the wrist, two fingers above the crease where wrist meets hand, that according to the traditions of acupuncture is the point that controls nausea. This, too, has been proven effective in scientific studies. Simple wrist bands with a bead sewn into them to provide pressure at this spot ("SeaBands" are one brand) have been used for years for seasickness; they are also effective for morning sickness. Similar battery-powered wrist bands provide a mild electrical stimulation to this point, also providing relief from nausea.

generations, while others have passed the rigors of scientific study. What works for your neighbor may not work for you, so keep trying until you find the one for you. If you cannot keep any foods or liquids down, or if you have lost more than a pound or two, be sure to let your doctor know.

If the measures in table 7.1 are ineffective, your doctor may prescribe anti-nausea medications by pill or rectal suppository. For cases of severe hyperemesis gravidarum, hospitalization is necessary to replace fluids and nutrients that are lost through almost constant vomiting. Sometimes you will be sent home with a special IV line to allow you to receive fluids and anti-nausea medication at home.

While morning sickness is never pleasant, you can at least take some comfort in the fact that you are not alone in experiencing it. Morning sickness is, the vast majority of the time, self-limited as well, all but disappearing by 13–14 weeks.

From My Journal

"You've been showing me your presence in the mornings—I gag after breakfast every morning and if I don't eat dinner by 6:30 or 7:00 I feel sick again. I'm not complaining—every time I retch I thank you for letting me know you are there."

Frequently Asked Questions

Q **The mere thought of taking my prenatal vitamins makes me gag. How important are they?**

A *Prenatal vitamins are like an insurance policy; if you eat a healthy diet (see week 11 for guidelines), you'll get most of what you need, but the vitamin provides a back-up for those days when a bite on the run is all you have time for. If you miss a couple of weeks of your vitamins, neither you nor the baby will suffer. Sometimes, changing a brand of vitamin or even taking it at a different time of day will allow you to keep it down. Some women find they can tolerate chewable vitamins; two Flintstones a day is an acceptable alternative. If you cannot tolerate your vitamin for now, don't sweat it, but try again in a few weeks when your nausea has lessened.*

Q I am so much sicker now than I was with my son, who is five. Does this mean I'm having a girl?

A *The old wives' tale is that girls make you sicker than boys, but there is no scientific evidence to back that up (this places it right up there in inaccuracy with another old wives' tale correlating the baby's heart rate with its gender!). Morning sickness results from a complex interplay between HCG levels, estrogen levels, gastrointestinal sensitivity, and psycho-social factors. Twins, on the other hand, are associated with more nausea and vomiting because HCG levels are significantly higher.*

Q I have blue lines on my breasts. What are they?

A *These blue lines snaking across your breasts are dilated veins. Your breasts are already working hard in preparation for feeding your baby several months down the line, and in order for glands to grow, blood supply to the breast must increase. These veins are much more prominent on fair-skinned women, and they will shrink (along with the newfound cleavage for those of us who are A-cups when not pregnant or lactating!) after pregnancy and nursing are complete.*

Q I have horrible morning—make that all day—sickness. I've lost 10 pounds and I can't even keep water down. I don't want to be hospitalized, so I haven't called my doctor. What should I do?

A *You do not have to suffer with morning sickness, but if you have tried all the remedies listed in Table 7.1, and you are losing weight, you must let your doctor know. If you become extremely dehydrated and malnourished, both you and your baby will suffer. You can develop electrolyte imbalances that can cause muscle weakness, liver dysfunction or even heart arrhythmias. Your baby may not grow properly if you have long-term nutritional deficiencies.*

If hospitalization is necessary, it is usually only for a few days, in order to rehydrate you and provide anti-nausea medications intravenously. Sometimes, IV feeding (called hyperalimentation) is necessary. If this is the case, a special long-term IV line is placed and you are discharged home. Home health nurses hook you up to the special nutritional IV fluids once a day, and IV medications can be given as well if you continue to vomit. Once you are feeling better and able to tolerate regular foods, therapy is stopped.

Week 8

SUN   DATE 10/14

MON   DATE 10/15

✗ TUE   DATE 10/9

WED   DATE 10/10

THUR   DATE 10/11

FRI   DATE 10/12

SAT   DATE 10/13

What Happened This Week?

Still light cramping - maybe related to bloating?

How I Feel Physically and Emotionally

g & I traveled to San Fran
Seems that I'm queezy all day if I get
up & going to fast

54

Dashed Hopes

Once you have reached this stage, about 80 percent of you will be able to breathe a sigh of relief that you will not miscarry. Unfortunately, about 20 percent of recognized pregnancies will end in miscarriage, and this number increases to 25 percent by age 40. Another 1–2 out of every 100 women reading this will have an *ectopic pregnancy*, one which develops outside the uterine cavity.

What Baby Is Doing

On ultrasound, babies as early as 8 weeks (6 weeks after fertilization) have been seen to make spontaneous twitching movements. Pigment is present in the retina, so the eye is very obvious, a dark spot on either side of baby's head. The external ear begins to form, as do the nose and upper lip. The head is still huge in relationship to the rest of the body and is still curled on the chest.

A bend in the arm is easily seen, and on the large, paddle-like hand plates, the beginning of fingers are forming. Fingers will remain webbed for a couple more weeks. Hand development precedes foot development by several days.

This week, the liver begins to produce red blood cells, taking over from the yolk sac. The pancreas and appendix are recognizable. Loops of the small intestine protrude into the umbilical cord at this stage because the bowel is growing more rapidly than the abdominal cavity can accommodate.

At the end of the eighth week, your baby is 13 mm long, measured from top of the head to bottom of its bottom (called the *crown–rump length,* CRL). This is about the size of a bay shrimp.

What You Are Doing

Your uterus is about the size of a grapefruit now, but it is still well below the pubic bone so you cannot feel it yet. You may, however, notice mild cramps similar to that "I'm about to get my period" feeling. This happens as the uterus grows and, if mild and not associated with spotting, is perfectly normal. If you have gained any weight at all, it should be minimal—no more than a pound or two.

Relaxin (a hormone secreted by the corpus luteum and the placenta) and other hormones lead to laxity of joints and tendons in pregnancy. This means that sudden shifts in direction (such as occur playing tennis, for example) may lead to injury more easily. Later in pregnancy, this loosening of the joints and

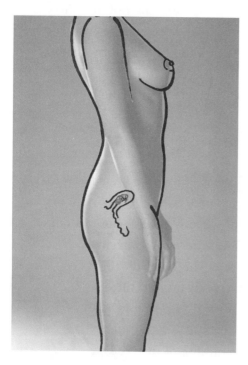

At 8 weeks, your outward appearance is little changed.

tendons is important, as it allows enough room for the baby to pass through the pelvis.

Special Considerations

When we get the positive result on the pregnancy test, we all hope for happy and healthy outcomes to our pregnancies, and for most of us, that is the case. For about 20 percent of us, however, that initial joy and excitement will be replaced by the sadness of a miscarriage or of finding out the pregnancy is developing outside the uterus (an ectopic pregnancy). These are important issues for older moms-to-be, because the incidence of miscarriage increases with age. While the overall miscarriage rate of recognized pregnancies is 20 percent, it ranges from about 12 percent in the 20-year-old to 25 percent in a 40-year-old woman. The majority of miscarriages—more than 50 percent—occur because of a chromosomal abnormality and (as will be discussed in detail in weeks 10 and 16) the chance of a chromosomal abnormality increases with age.

If you have had a miscarriage before, you are probably worried that it will happen again. One miscarriage does not increase the chance of a second. You may also be worried that something you are doing—or not doing—may cause a miscarriage. Rest assured, with a few exceptions, nothing

> ## ✎ DOCTOR'S NOTES
>
> I am well aware of all aspects of miscarriage, not only because I am an ob-gyn and almost every week of the year have to take care of women who miscarry, but also because I have had three miscarriages myself—two before my daughter was born and the third while I was writing this book. I understand the physical and emotional pain, the sense of loss, and the feeling of failure that can accompany a miscarriage.

you do or don't do will make you lose your baby. Women who smoke, use street drugs (especially cocaine), or drink moderately or heavily do have a higher chance of miscarrying, but that margarita you had before you even knew you were pregnant or those 3 days of prenatal vitamins you forgot to take or that hike in the mountains will not cause a miscarriage.

What happens when a woman miscarries? Some will notice spotting or bleeding like a period; often this is associated with pretty significant cramping. Others will not spot or bleed, but will call saying they just do not feel pregnant any more. Some women will get the bad news on the basis of a routine ultrasound, when the heartbeat is not seen. Depending on how far along you are, and, if you are already bleeding, how heavy the bleeding is, you may be given the options of miscarrying on your own or having a *D&C*. This surgical procedure involves *dilating* the cervix and then *curretting*, or scraping, the walls of the uterus to remove the pregnancy. There are good and bad points to either approach, and the decision is between you and your doctor.

A miscarriage is a loss, and losses deserve to be mourned.

> ### From My Journal
>
> "I hope this time works. I really want to be your mom—and Jeff wants to be your dad. He is excited, in a subdued "We've been through this before only to be disappointed" way. We love you already and are waiting for you with open arms. Please stay with us this time. . . . Please take root and grow in me. I will do my best to nurture you and provide a home for the 9 months. I will try not to let fear close my heart to you—don't for a minute think I am afraid of you—I am afraid of losing you. I want you to be my child, more than anything."

Friends, acquaintances, and family members may try to tell you "It's for the best," or "You can get pregnant again." Yes, you probably can get pregnant again, but it won't be *that* baby. Allow yourself the time and the space you need to grieve, and try to surround yourself with understanding and supportive people. If you feel depressed after a miscarriage, you are not abnormal and you are not alone—when interviewed six months later, 50 percent of women who miscarried were found to be clinically depressed.

An ectopic pregnancy is one in which the baby develops outside the uterine cavity, most commonly in one of the fallopian tubes. This happens because the tubes have been damaged in the past, either from infection (commonly, an STD like chlamydia) or endometriosis. The pregnancy can grow for several weeks, but cannot survive and cannot be transplanted into the uterus in order to continue development until birth. Growth will occur until a certain point, and then the tube can stretch no further; it may then rupture, leading to a potentially life-threatening internal hemorrhage.

Classically, an ectopic pregnancy is diagnosed on the basis of spotting in early pregnancy associated with one-sided pain. Blood HCG levels may be abnormal, usually because the levels do not rise appropriately over the course of several days. An ultrasound may reveal a mass in one of the tubes, or just the lack of a visible pregnancy within the uterus.

Ectopic pregnancies are ob-gyn emergencies and require immediate evaluation and intervention. Traditionally, surgery was done and the tube with the ectopic pregnancy was removed. Today, if detected early enough, medical management with *methotrexate* may be effective, and surgery may be avoided. Methotrexate is a form of chemotherapy that leads to re-absorbtion of the pregnancy. If methotrexate is not an option, minimally invasive laparoscopic techniques may allow surgery to be performed through a few tiny incisions, and the abnormally located pregnancy tissue may be removed without taking the entire tube.

Frequently Asked Questions

Q I am having a sharp pain in my left side. I have had an ectopic pregnancy on the right before and lost that tube. Because of damage to my left tube, I underwent IVF, so the embryo was placed directly into my uterus. There's no way this could be another ectopic, right? So what could this pain be?

A *This pain could be an ovarian cyst, even just a corpus luteum cyst. It could be scar tissue from prior infection, endometriosis, or surgery. It could even be a left-sided tubal pregnancy—IVF (in vitro fertilization) does not guarantee that a pregnancy will be in the proper location. Ectopics are less common with IVF, but they do occur—I've seen two in my career. When the embryos are transferred into the uterine cavity, they may be injected with enough force to cause one or more to enter the tube. If this embryo implants, an ectopic is the result.*

With pain on one side and a history of a prior ectopic, you will need to contact your doctor. Blood HCG levels will be drawn and an ultrasound ordered. A series of blood tests over the course of several days and one or more ultrasounds may be required before an ectopic pregnancy is ruled in or ruled out.

Q I have been diagnosed with a "missed abortion" at 8 weeks, and the doctor said I could have a D&C or wait to miscarry on my own. I don't know what to do! And what is a missed abortion?

A *Missed abortion is a term from the days before ultrasounds were so routine. It refers to a pregnancy that stopped developing at some point and has yet to miscarry after several weeks. Today, we use this term to describe a situation where an early ultrasound does not show a heartbeat when it should, yet no significant bleeding or cramping have occurred.*

Most early pregnancy losses will miscarry on their own prior to 8–10 weeks; after that, a D&C is usually recommended due to the excessive bleeding that may accompany a later miscarriage. Some women want to "get it over with" and choose a D&C on emotional grounds. D&Cs are not without risks, however, although the incidence of complications is low. These risks include introduction of infection, uterine perforation, and scarring of the uterine cavity that may affect the ability to conceive or carry a pregnancy in the future. Allowing Mother Nature to take her course carries the risk of hemorrhage and the need for an emergency D&C.

Everyone's desires and situation are different, and often whether or not to have a D&C is not so much a matter of which choice is better from a medical standpoint, but which is better for you emotionally. I wish this was a question that no one would ever have to face.

✎ DOCTOR'S NOTES

I have had three miscarriages—with #1 and #3, I had a D&C, but with # 2 I waited to miscarry on my own. Neither way was pleasant. I chose the D&Cs because with #1, I was more than 8 weeks pregnant and didn't want to start bleeding heavily when I was doing surgery or on call and with #3, I was about to go out of town for a medical meeting and didn't want to have to go to a strange emergency room in the middle of the night, plus I had my 18-month-old daughter to think about. With #2, my blighted ovum (a fertilized egg that just never goes anywhere) was diagnosed at 6 weeks, and I felt the odds of heavy bleeding were low.

Week 9

SUN   DATE 10/21

MON   DATE 10/22

TUE   DATE 10/16

WED   DATE 10/17

THUR   DATE 10/18

FRI   DATE 10/19

SAT   DATE 10/20

What Happened This Week?

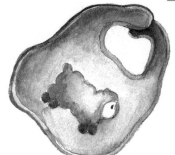

How I Feel Physically and Emotionally

Teratogens, or What to Avoid When You're Expecting

WHILE YOUR BABY is generally well protected in the intrauterine environment, there are substances that can cross the placenta and harm the developing child. *Teratogens* are any substances or factors that can cause permanent alterations in the form or function of a baby. Because most of the major organ systems are developing between weeks 5 and 10, this is the time when the baby is most vulnerable.

What Baby Is Doing

Changes this week are most pronounced in the arms and legs. Fingers, although short and webbed, are clearly visible. The beginning of toes can be seen as well. At this point, the wrists and ankles are still fused with the hands and feet. The skeleton is mainly cartilage, but bone formation is beginning in the arms. Knees and elbows bend, and the baby can be seen to "wave" on ultrasound.

The eyelids have formed, although they will remain fused shut for many more weeks. The external ear is well formed. The neck is better developed, so the head no longer lays right on the chest. The yolk sac begins to deteriorate, as the liver is now producing red blood cells and the placenta is taking over the job of transporting nutrients and oxygen from mom to baby, and waste products from baby to you.

The lungs are continuing to branch and all the bronchi are now present. In the intestinal tract, the duodenum is now hollow and the stomach acids can empty into the small intestine.

Your baby is now 18 mm long, about the size of a cashew nut. Occasionally, the heartbeat may be heard with a *doppler*.

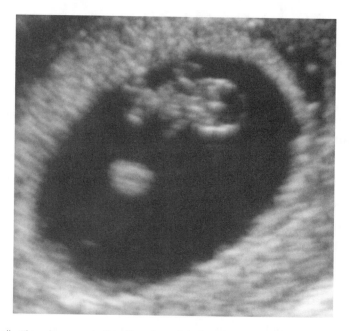

"Spacewalk. This ultrasound of an 8 to 9 week baby reminds me of astronauts in space. The baby's head, large in proportion to the rest of the body, is on the right. Two tiny arms and two tiny legs can be seen sticking out from the body. The gray circle beneath the baby is the yolk sac."

What You Are Doing

You still look pretty much the same as you did before your little passenger came on board. Your breasts are probably larger and your waistline may not be quite as well defined, but you still do not look obviously pregnant. Some women do "glow" when pregnant due to increased blood flow to the skin, but others may feel as if they are experiencing puberty once again with annoying breakouts.

Increases in blood volume really begin at this point; by the end of pregnancy, your blood plasma volume will have increased about 2.5 times! This increase in plasma volume is accompanied by an increased amount of fluid in cells throughout your body. Many women notice visual changes during pregnancy as the shape of the eyeball changes from this fluid; this seems to be especially pronounced in women who wear contact lenses. Occasionally a prescription change may be needed to ensure crisp vision.

From My Journal
"5/6/98 (9 weeks). Didn't have the usual post-break-fast retching this morning, so I was paranoid—went back to the office after doing a postpartum tubal and I HEARD YOUR HEART-BEAT!!!!!! It is the most beautiful, melodious sound. Brought the doppler home so Jeff can listen. . . . "

And I still get teary-eyed with couples in my office when we hear the heartbeat for the first time.

Special Considerations

In the population as a whole, about 3 percent of babies will be noted to have a major birth defect; this number has not changed in eons and will probably remain in the 3 percent range forever. More than half the time, a reason for the birth defect cannot be found. In other cases, exposure to certain substances, infections, or physical agents is identified as the cause. Right after fertilization, exposure to teratogens usually produces an all-or-none effect: the exposure is so great that it causes a miscarriage, or it has no impact at all.

After the embryonic stage, exposure can still cause abnormalities, but it may be limited to poor growth of the baby or a particular organ or to some functional impairment, rather than gross structural abnormalities.

While many women fear things they have been exposed to, the list of proven teratogens is actually quite small (see table 9.1 for a partial list). The effect a given agent may have depends not only on when in pregnancy the exposure occurred, but also the duration of exposure and the genetic susceptibility of the baby. One example of the differing effects of exposure at different points in pregnancy is chicken pox: If you contract chicken pox in the first 16 weeks of pregnancy, there is a 20 percent chance that your baby could develop scarring of the skin, incomplete development of the fingers and toes, eye damage, and mental retardation; after 20 weeks, however, there is no risk of such birth defects.

While only 7–10 percent of birth defects can be attributed to known teratogens, the best advice is to avoid using any prescription, over-the-counter, or recreational drug (including alcohol) during the first trimester. Vitamins other than prenatals and herbs should be avoided as well, unless you have gotten your doctor's explicit okay. What if you must take a prescription medication for a chronic condition? Ideally, you had a preconception visit with your doctor and have been placed on the safest medication; sometimes the benefit to you outweighs any potential risks to the baby (some anti-seizure medications are good examples of this—the seizures themselves probably cause more harm to a developing baby than do the medications). What if you took an over-the-counter medication for a cold before you realized you were pregnant? Be sure to let your doctor know what it was and when you took it—in all likelihood, there will be no harm done. Commonly used medications like ace-

TABLE 9.1

Known Teratogens (Partial List)

ACE Inhibitors

Enalapril, captopril, blood pressure medications

Kidney abnormalities, poor growth, and low birthweight.

Alcohol

Mental retardation, poor growth pre- and post-birth, abnormal facial features, heart defects, kidney defects. Women who drink 6 drinks per day have a 40 percent chance of delivering a baby with fetal alcohol syndrome. Lesser amounts may cause varying degrees of abnormality (called *fetal alcohol effect*). We do not know if any level of alcohol consumption is "safe."

Carbamezapine

Tegretol, an anti-seizure drug

Neural tube defects (e.g., spina bifida), poor growth. Risk of spina bifida is only 1 percent, higher if used along with other anti-seizure medications. Exposure after the sixth week, when the neural tube has closed, cannot cause spina bifida.

Coumadin

Warfarin, a blood thinner

Small nose, bone abnormalities, poor growth, eye defects. Risk is 15–20 percent when used in the first trimester. Later exposure can increase the risk of placental abruption or bleeding in the baby.

Cocaine

Incomplete development of the bowel, malformations of the heart, face, limbs and genitourinary tract, strokes, mental retardation. Placental abruption and stillbirth are not uncommon.

TABLE 9.1

Cytomegalovirus (CMV)

Hydrocephalus ("water on the brain"), eye damage, mental retardation, hearing loss, poor growth. If mom contracts CMV for the first time while pregnant, especially in the 1st trimester, 40 percent of babies will become infected; of those babies, 20 percent will have the above birth defects.

Lead

Increase in miscarriage and stillbirths. Preconception lead level determination should be performed for those at risk due to occupational exposure or living in an older dwelling, where lead-based paint may have been used.

Lithium

For bipolar disorder

Ebstein anomaly, a heart defect. Risk is low.

Mercury

Mental retardation, seizures, blindness, cerebral palsy.

Phenytoin

Dilantin, an anti-seizure drug

Poor growth, mental retardation, small head, abnormal facial features, heart defects. The full syndrome affects <10 percent of babies exposed. As with Carbamazepine, the effect of untreated seizures may be worse.

Rubella (German Measles)

Small head and brain, mental retardation, cataracts, deafness. Half of all babies exposed to rubella in the first trimester will have some degree of malformations; this drops to 6 percent if infection occurs after the twentieth week.

TABLE 9.1

Tetracycline

Antibiotic

Yellow-brown discoloration of teeth ONLY if taken in the second or third trimester; no effect if taken early in pregnancy.

Toxoplasmosis

Small head and brain, mental retardation, eye damage. Risk to baby only if mom contracts the infection for the first time during pregnancy. Birth defects are most severe if toxoplasmosis is contracted during the first trimester, although risk of infection passing to the baby is only about 10 percent with first-trimester exposure.

Valproic Acid

Anti-seizure medication

Neural tube defects (especially spina bifida). See Carbamazepine.

Varicella (Chicken Pox)

Cataracts, skin scarring, small head, incomplete development of the hands and feet. Infection after 20 weeks does not cause any of these malformations. Infection with chicken pox within 5 to 7 days of delivery, however, can lead to the baby developing chicken pox at birth.

Vitamin A Derivatives

Accutane

Increased rate of miscarriage, cleft lip and palate, small eyes, small or missing ears, other facial abnormalities, central nervous system defects, heart defects. Topical preparations like Retin-A do not cause any problems.

X-rays

Mental retardation, small head. Less than 5 rads causes no harm whatsoever; most x-rays (chest x-ray, IVP, etc.) deliver < 1 rad.

tominophen (Tylenol), antihistamines (Sudafed), and cough suppressants (Robitussin) are generally considered safe.

In addition to your doctor, there are several excellent resources for information on possible teratogens. The Organization of Teratogen Information Services (*www.otis.org*) is a clearinghouse for information, organized by geographic regions. In the eastern United States call:

Massachusetts Teratogen Information Service
Boston, MA
617-466-8474

and in the western United States call:

Pregnancy Riskline
Salt Lake City, UT
801-328-2229

Frequently Asked Questions

Q My fortieth birthday was, as it turns out, 5 days after I conceived. My husband threw a wild surprise party for me and I had a few too many drinks. Could I have hurt my baby?

A *No, you did no harm to your baby by having a wild time on your fortieth birthday. First, as you may recall from week 3, implantation does not occur until 6–7 days after fertilization; prior to implantation, there is no connection between you and the baby, and therefore substances you ingest, like alcohol, cannot get to the baby. Second, even if implantation had occurred, there is no evidence that a drink or two on rare occasions will cause any harm. Now that you know you are pregnant, however, avoid alcohol in the first trimester.*

Q I have high blood pressure and am on an ACE inhibitor. I know I shouldn't be on this type of medicine while pregnant, and my doctor's appointment isn't for another 2 weeks. Should I just stop now?

A *Do not stop your medication prior to talking to your doctor because your blood pressure may skyrocket without treatment, and this is not good for you or the baby. It is true that ACE inhibitors are not recommended during pregnancy, but their adverse effects (poor growth, decreased amniotic fluid, and poor kidney function) occur with exposure later in pregnancy. Use of ACE inhibitors in the first trimester has not been associated with any significant risk to the baby.*

Your doctor will change your medication to one that is safer in pregnancy. Methyldopa (Aldomet) is the anti-hypertensive that has been used most extensively in pregnancy and is thought to be the

✎ DOCTOR'S NOTES

Many of my patients ask me about an occasional drink during pregnancy. My advice is this: No alcohol in the first trimester. After that, an occasional glass of wine or beer on a special occasion (birthday, anniversary, New Year's Eve) is okay—but every day is not a special occasion! I personally did not drink one drop of alcohol from the moment I conceived (I was on fertility drugs and had an insemination so I knew exactly when that was) until after I delivered. My husband and I are wine collectors and we have a wonderful cellar of some pretty darn good wines; he'd be drinking a '94 Opus One and I'd have lemonade with dinner! While I love a good glass of cabernet, it was not worth it to me to drink while I was pregnant, and, in fact, I had no desire to drink in the first place.

safest. Other anti-hypertensives (like beta blockers or calcium channel blockers) may be continued if you are on them prior to pregnancy; again, your doctor will discuss which medication is best for you and your baby.

Q I was not planning on becoming pregnant. In fact, I was using birth control pills! I was on them for almost 2 months before I found out I was pregnant. Will this cause birth defects?

A *Birth control pills, as you found out, are not 100 percent reliable. There is a risk of genital abnormalities in female fetuses exposed to synthetic progesterone. Masculinization of the genitals occurs in 0.3 percent; most of this information is derived from exposure to medroxyprogesterone acetate (Provera), sometimes used to bring on a period, rather than from the types of synthetic progesterone in birth control pills. Current thinking is that the risk of a birth defect from the Pill is not different than the background risk of birth defects in the first place and no special testing need be done. Many women who conceive on the Pill, however, will need an early ultrasound to determine their due date because they will have no idea when they may have conceived!*

Q I have heartburn like you won't believe. I can't sleep, I'm miserable. What can I do about it? And, is it true that this means the baby will be born with lots of hair?

A *The heartburn-hair connection is one of those old wives' tales that cannot be laid to rest! You are as likely to deliver a baldy as you are to deliver a baby who needs his first haircut before he leaves the hospital.*

There are ways to diminish the distress of heartburn. First, avoid eating heavy, greasy, or overly spicy foods. Second, eat smaller amounts at a time. The reason you have heartburn is that your stomach cannot digest food as efficiently; relaxation of the junction be-

tween stomach and esophagus means digestive acids can more easily backwash into the esophagus, producing that uncomfortable burning sensation. If you put less into your stomach at a time, you will be less likely to have acid reflux. Third, stay upright for a couple of hours after eating, again to prevent acid reflux. You may even need to sleep propped up. And, finally, use antacids when necessary. I am a fan of Tums, because not only do they help neutralize stomach acids, they provide calcium, too.

Week 10

SUN _____ DATE 10/28

MON _____ DATE 10/29

✗ TUE _____ DATE 10/23

WED _____ DATE 10/24

THUR _____ DATE 10/25

FRI _____ DATE 10/26

SAT _____ DATE 10/27

What Happened This Week?

_____

_____

_____

_____

How I Feel Physically and Emotionally

_____

_____

_____

_____

Chorionic Villus Sampling

WHILE WE ARE all individuals, and some of us will have complications while others will sail through pregnancy with nary a hitch, we are all at increased risk of having a baby with a chromosomal abnormality. Because we have passed (or will pass by the time of delivery) the magic age of 35, we are considered of "advanced maternal age." Genetic testing is available to determine whether the baby you are carrying has a chromosomal defect, but only you can decide whether you wish to avail yourself of the testing and what you will do with the information it provides.

What Baby Is Doing

This marks the beginning of the final week of the embryonic stage; after this week, your baby is officially known as a *fetus* until birth. Fingers become distinct this week, and the webbing between them disappears; toes become separate a few days later than the fingers. The tail, so prominent a few weeks ago, is a mere stub early this week, and will disappear completely by the beginning of the eleventh week. Your baby looks distinctly human at this point.

The anal membrane has broken down, so the gastrointestinal tract is open from the mouth to the anus. Although external genitalia are still not differentiated (boys and girls look the same at this point), testosterone secretion has begun in boys.

✎ DOCTOR'S NOTES

Don't ask me why I keep using foodstuffs as analogies for the size of your baby. Maybe it is because I am a woman and I take my ruler and go into my kitchen to see what is 10 or 30 or 50 mm in size!

By the end of the tenth week, your baby is about 3 cm (1.2 in) long, from crown to rump. This is the size of a pitted prune. If, and I stress *if*, you are lucky (and thin and your uterus is not tilted backward), your baby's heartbeat *may* be heard with a doppler.

What You Are Doing

You still don't need to run out and buy maternity clothes, although you may not be able to button your favorite pair of jeans anymore! (Hint: Wear shirts tucked out and loop a rubber band through the button hole and around the button—no one will ever know!) The corpus luteum is still churning out progesterone, but not for much longer; the placenta will completely take over that function during the next two weeks.

You may notice irregular brownish patches on your face or neck; called *chloasma,* or the "mask of pregnancy," this is caused by markedly elevated levels of melanocyte stimulating hormone from about the eighth week on. This is also responsible for the *linea nigra,* a dark line from breastbone to pubic bone which often appears as well. Both of these pigment changes fade after delivery.

At this point in your pregnancy, you may have gained a few pounds. The total average weight of baby, placenta, amniotic fluid, increased breast tissue, blood volume, uterus, and fat is only 23 ounces!

Special Considerations

As I've said before (here and to my patients), I'd much rather take care of a healthy, motivated 39-year-old than an obese, smoking, couch potato 25-year-old. Even with the added risks of age, an older woman in good general health is likely to have a better pregnancy and a healthier baby than a younger woman who does not take care of herself or her unborn baby. Good habits, however, can only go so far, and no matter how wonderful a shape you are in, you can do nothing about the biologic fact that your eggs are older. This translates into an increased risk of having a baby with a chromosomal abnormality that is directly linked to your age (see table 10.1).

While your doctor cannot change the chromosomes you pass on to your baby, she can offer testing to see if your baby is chromosomally normal or not. Two of the tests currently available are *chorionic villus sampling* (CVS) and *amniocentesis*. These tests cannot, however, pick up every defect; we can only look for abnormalities in the baby's genetic structure that we have learned to identify. These tests cannot predict mental capacity nor detect problems like cleft lip or extra toes. There is no test or combination of tests that can guarantee a perfectly normal outcome. As mentioned in week 9, the background risk of birth defects is about 3 percent, and this number has not changed, nor is it expected to change, despite all the advances in technology.

Chorionic villus sampling is done between the tenth and twelfth weeks of pregnancy and will be discussed there. Amniocentesis is done after 14–15 weeks (most commonly at 16 weeks) and will be discussed in week 16. Remember, both of these tests, along with a

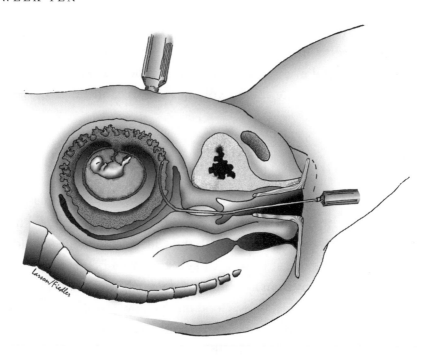

During CVS, a long thin catheter is passed through the cervix and into the developing placenta (on the front wall of the uterus in this illustration).

blood test called AFP (alph fetoprotein), should always be offered to you, but the decision whether to have them or not is up to you only. Your doctor should discuss the risks and benefits with you, but she should not force her personal opinions on you.

CVS is a technique that has been performed since the early 1970s, but was not widely available until the mid- to late 1980s. With CVS, a small sample of the placenta is obtained via a catheter placed through the cervix (most common) or through the abdominal and uterine walls. Because the chorionic villi of the placenta are of fetal origin, this tissue reflects the chromosomal status of the baby. Both ways of performing CVS are done under direct ultrasound visualization. CVS should only be performed by doctors who have extensive experience with the technique; general ob-gyns do not usually perform CVS, but will refer you to a *perinatologist* or *geneticist* who has been well trained in the techniques.

TABLE 10.1

Incidence of Chromosomal Abnormalities by Maternal Age at Time of Delivery

Age	Down Syndrome	Any Chromosomal Abnormality
15	1:1578	1:454
20	1:1528	1:525
25	1:1351	1:475
30	1:909	1:384
35	1:384	1:178
36	1:307	1:148
37	1:242	1:122
38	1:189	1:104
39	1:146	1:80
40	1:112	1:62
41	1:85	1:48
42	1:65	1:38
43	1:49	1:30
44	1:37	1:23
45	1:28	1:18
46	1:21	1:14
47	1:15	1:10
48	1:11	1:8
49	1:8	1:6
50	1:6	N/A

✎ DOCTOR'S NOTES

I was 37 when I conceived my daughter, to turn 38 three weeks prior to her due date. I elected to have CVS done. I chose an excellent specialist about 2 hours from my home. Even though I am an ob-gyn, my husband and I were counseled for 45 minutes before the test was performed. The procedure itself was absolutely painless in my case, although some women will experience cramps and spotting. I thought it was so cool to watch the catheter pick up the chorionic villi, but my husband just held my hand and tried not to look at anything! A little more than 24 hours later I got a phone call from the nurse, informing me the preliminary results showed we were having a chromosomally normal girl!

Once the chorionic villi are obtained, and they are successfully obtained in 99.7 percent of women, they are analyzed to determine the baby's chromosomal, or DNA, status. Because these cells grow rapidly, test results are available in a relatively short period of time—1–2 days for preliminary results and 7–10 days for the final results. CVS cannot, however, be used to detect neural tube defects (e.g., spina bifida); if CVS is performed, a blood AFP should be drawn at 16 weeks (see week 15 for more information on AFP testing).

CVS is considered a relatively safe test. When done between 10 and 12 weeks, the risk of miscarriage as a result of the test is about 1 percent. This is slightly higher than that associated with amniocentesis, the trade-off for having results significantly earlier in the pregnancy. CVS also may increase the risk of the baby being born with missing fingertips or toes; a study conducted by the CDC estimated this risk to be 1:3,000, but in an international study this did not occur in any greater number than in the general population not undergoing CVS.

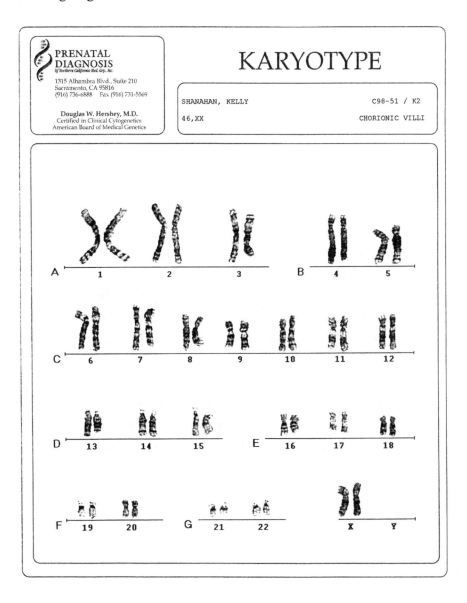

Frequently Asked Questions

Q My doctor told me I'm at increased risk for a baby with a chromosomal abnormality because I will be 36 when I give birth. Why is that?

A *The egg you ovulated and that was fertilized contributed its DNA to what is now your baby. That egg and that DNA have been present since before you were born. In almost 37 years (the 36 since you have been born and the 9 months before that) there has been much opportunity for damage. The egg, before ovulation, contains 46 chromosomes (two of each of the 23 different chromosomes all humans have). Just prior to ovulation, one chromosome out of each pair is discarded, so that the egg contains 23 chromosomes. Sometimes—and with increasing frequency with age—this does not happen properly and a pair of chromosomes will remain joined. When fertilization occurs and the sperm contributes its 23 chromosomes, the resultant baby will have an extra chromosome, derived from mom. Down syndrome (AKA Trisomy 21, meaning there are three, rather than the normal two, copies of chromosome #21) is the most common example of this. See table 10.1 for the incidence of chromosomal abnormalities by age.*

Q I know I'm more likely to have a baby with Down syndrome because I am 40, and I know that Down syndrome involves mental retardation, but I'm not really sure what else it means.

A *Down syndrome, occurs when a baby has an extra chromosome 21; the medical name for Down syndrome is Trisomy 21, meaning there are 3 copies of the twenty-first chromosome. This extra chromosome 21 leads to varying degrees of mental retardation and a characteristic appearance: sloping forehead; flat nasal bridge; eyes that appear widely spaced due to exaggerated* epicanthal folds; *protruding tongue; short, stubby fingers; a single, rather than the usual two, crease in the palm of the hand. There are heart defects in 30–40 percent of children with Down syndrome.*

The degree of mental retardation cannot be predicted by any form of genetic testing. Most people with Down syndrome fall in the category of mild mental retardation, with an IQ between 60 and 70 (100 is an average IQ), and most will eventually be able to work and live semi-independently. Children with Down syndrome are often very happy and lovable, described by others as "sunny."

Q My doctor mentioned CVS or amniocentesis as options for genetic testing. Why is one better than the other?

A *CVS is not better than amniocentesis, or vice versa; they are both options, each with their own pluses and minuses. One of the major advantages of CVS is that it is done earlier in the pregnancy, so you know if there is a chromosomal problem or not while you are in your first trimester.*

Q I would not have an abortion under any circumstances. Why would my doctor even offer genetic testing to me?

A *It is not for your doctor or anyone else to decide whether you should terminate a chromosomally abnormal baby or not. It is your doctor's duty to inform you that genetic testing is available. Many women would never think about aborting a baby, even if they knew the baby would have birth defects, but they want to know ahead of time so they can learn about the condition and find out what resources are available in their community to ensure the best possible chances for that child after birth. Some women would rather just wait and see what happens, finding out about an abnormality, even if it is one that is incompatible with life outside the uterus, at the time of birth. Other women know that they do not have what it takes to care for a child with special needs. The decision to have genetic testing— or not—and the decision as to what to do with such information if testing is performed, is up to you, and only you.*

Week 11

SUN   DATE 1/4

MON   DATE 1/5

✗ TUE   DATE 10/30

WED   DATE 10/31

THUR   DATE 11/1

FRI   DATE 11/2

SAT   DATE 11/3

What Happened This Week?

How I Feel Physically and Emotionally

Eating for Two

THERE'S AN OLD 10,000 Maniacs song, "I eat for two, walk for two, breathe for two now," and while yes, you are eating for two, that does not mean you eat twice as much. Quantity takes a definite backseat to quality when it comes to nutrition in pregnancy.

What Baby Is Doing

At this point, the baby's head accounts for half of the crown–rump length. Rapid growth in the body will occur over the next three weeks, but your baby's head will appear disproportionate to its body even after birth. The eyes are widely spaced and the ears are set low on the head. The legs are short in relationship to the rest of the body.

At 11 weeks, the liver, churning out red blood cells, accounts for 10 percent of the baby's total weight. The kidneys begin to function, and urine is produced. This urine will eventually make up the bulk of the amniotic fluid. Waste products from the baby are transported across the placenta into your body's circulation and are disposed of by you.

By the end of this week, the average baby is 50 mm (5 cm, or 2 in) long, about the size of an apricot. Your baby tips the scale at 8 gm (0.3 ounces).

What You Are Doing

You are probably still tired, still nauseated, and still not showing. Be patient—all of these things will change over the next few weeks! On a pelvic exam, your uterus is obviously enlarged to the size of a cantaloupe (there's that fruit analogy again!).

Starting this week and continuing until about 25 weeks, there is a rapid rise in plasma volume, the amount of fluid in the vascular system. This contributes to a gradual decline in *hemoglobin* due to dilution; average hemoglobin pre-pregnancy is about 13 gm/dl (grams per deciliter), and this decreases to an average of 11 gm/dl at term. Anemia of pregnancy contributes to fatigue. By this point you will probably also have noticed that your heart rate has increased by about 15 beats per minute. Some palpitations are normal, although severely irregular or very rapid heart beats, especially if accompanied by significant shortness of breath, should be reported to your doctor.

Special Considerations

"Eating for two" is something your grandmother told your mother, and your mother told you, but somewhere in the translation, women have developed the misperception that pregnancy is a time when you can eat whatever—and as much—as you want. Nothing could be further from the truth. Your baby is completely and utterly dependent on you for all its needs, and proper nutrition and adequate weight gain can ensure the best possible start in life. A couple of studies—one done years ago and another more recently—have shown that 95 percent of women whose diets were excellent gave birth to babies in excellent health, whereas 65 percent of women whose diets were largely made up of junk foods delivered premature, stillborn, or unhealthy babies.

What you eat and the weight you gain has implications for both the short- and long-term health of your child. Poor nutrition increases the chance of prematurity, low birthweight, *pre-eclampsia*, and stillbirth. Also, moms who do not get adequate amounts of protein are more likely to have children who will later develop high blood pressure.

Food Guide Pyramid
A Guide to Daily Food Choices

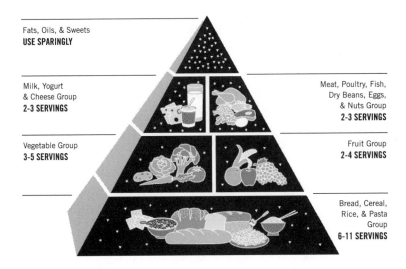

Fats, Oils, & Sweets
USE SPARINGLY

Milk, Yogurt & Cheese Group
2-3 SERVINGS

Meat, Poultry, Fish, Dry Beans, Eggs, & Nuts Group
2-3 SERVINGS

Vegetable Group
3-5 SERVINGS

Fruit Group
2-4 SERVINGS

Bread, Cereal, Rice, & Pasta Group
6-11 SERVINGS

In this first trimester, you do not need to consume 1 calorie more than you did 11 weeks ago, and for the remainder of your pregnancy, you only need an extra 250–300 calories per day. That is (as I run down to my kitchen again!) 1 container of low-fat yogurt and a small banana. So, now that I've burst your bubble about "eating for two" and you're wondering what to do about those pints of

TABLE 11.1

Grow-a-Healthy-Baby Foods

Whole Grains and Complex Carbohydrates (4–5 servings)

Black-eyed peas, 2/3 cup

Brown rice, 1/2 cup

Brown rice cakes, 2

Lentils, 1/2 cup

Oatmeal, 1 cup

Popcorn, 2 cups

Pinto, kidney, garbanzo, or black beans, 1/2 cup

Tortilla, 1

Wild rice, 1/2 cup

Whole grain cereal, 1 oz.

Whole wheat bagel, 1/2

Whole wheat bread, 1 slice

Whole wheat English muffin, 1/2

Whole wheat pasta, 1 oz. uncooked

Fruits and Vegetables (4–6 servings)

Apple, 1 medium

Apricots, 2 medium

Asparagus, 10 spears

Banana, 1 small

Blackberries, raspberries, boysenberries, 1 1/2 cups

Blueberries, 1 1/2 cups

Broccoli, 1/2 cup

Canteloupe, 1/4

Carrots, 1/2 small

Cauliflower, 2/3 cup

Corn, 1 small ear

TABLE 11.1

Fruits and Vegetables (continued)

Grapefruit, 1/2

Grapefruit or orange juice, 1/2 cup

Grapes, 2/3 cup

Green bell pepper, 1/2 medium

Honeydew melon, 1/8

Kale, mustard greens or chard, 3/4 cup cooked

Lettuce, 1 1/2 cups

Mango, 1/2

Orange, 1 small

Peach, 1 medium

Pear, 1 medium

Peas, 1 1/2 cups

Pineapple, 3/4 cup

Red bell pepper, 1/3 medium

Spinach, 1/2 cup raw or 1/4 cup cooked

Strawberries, 1/2 cup

Sweet potato, baked, 1/2 small

Tomatoes, 2 small

Tomato paste or puree, 1/2 cup

Tomato sauce, 1 1/4 cups

Vegetable juice, 3/4 cups

Watermelon, 2 cups

White potato, 1 small

Winter squash, mashed, 1/2 cup

Zucchini, 1/2 cup

TABLE 11.1

Protein (4 servings)

Almonds or walnuts, 3 oz.

Cheddar cheese, 3.5 oz.

Chicken or turkey, white meat, skinless, 2.5 oz.

Chicken or turkey, dark meat, skinless 3 oz.

Eggs, whites, 5

Eggs, whole, 2

Fresh fish, 3.5 oz.

Lamb, 3.5 oz.

Lean beef, 3 oz.

Lean pork, 3 oz.

Low-fat yogurt, 1 3/4 cups

Low-fat cottage cheese, 3/4 cup

Mozzarella cheese, 3 oz.

Nonfat milk, 2.5–3 8 oz. glasses

Oysters (cooked only!), 15–20

Peanut butter, 5 Tbsp.

Scallops, 4 oz.

Shrimp, 3.5 oz.

Sunflower seeds, 3.5 oz.

Swiss cheese, 3 oz.

Tofu, 5 oz.

Tuna, packed in water, 1 can

Calcium-Rich Foods (4 servings)

Almonds, 3/4 cup

Broccoli, fresh, 1 3/4 cups

Canned salmon with bones, 4 oz.

Canned sardines, with bones, 3 oz.

TABLE 11.1

Calcium-Rich Foods (continued)

Cheddar, provolone, or mozzarella, 1 1/2 oz.

Kale or turnip greens, cooked, 1 1/2 cups

Low-fat cottage cheese, 1 3/4 cups

Low-fat yogurt, 1 cup

Nonfat milk, 1 cup

Swiss cheese, 1 1/4 oz.

Tofu, 9 oz.

High-Fat Foods (2 servings)

Avocado, 1/2 small

Butter or margarine, 1 Tbsp.

Cream, 3 Tbsp.

Cream cheese, 2 Tbsp.

Mayonnaise, 1 Tbsp.

Peanut butter, 2 Tbsp.

Polyunsaturated vegetable oil (safflower, olive, canola), 1 Tbsp.

Sour cream, 4 Tbsp.

Whipping cream, 2 Tbsp.

premium ice cream in your freezer, what should you eat when pregnant? The answer is a well-rounded diet consisting of whole grains, fresh fruits and vegetables, high quality protein, calcium-rich foods, and modest amounts of unsaturated fats. In general, you should try to consume 4–5 servings of complex carbohydrates; 4–6 servings of fruits and vegetables; 4 servings of protein; 4 servings of calcium-rich foods; and only 2 high-fat items. Table 11.1 shows a list of such foods and approximate amounts for each serving. As you can see, some foods meet more than 1

TABLE 11.2

Recommended Daily Allowances

	Non-pregnant Woman	Pregnant Woman
Folate (mcg)	180	400
Niacin (mg)	15	17
Calcium (mg)	1000	1200
Iodine (mcg)	150	175
Iron (mg of ferrous iron)	15	30
Magnesium (mg)	280	320
Phosphorous (mg)	1200	1200
Protein (gm)	55	60
Riboflavin (mg)	1.3	1.6
Thiamine (mg)	1.1	1.5
Vitamin A (mcg)	800	800
Vitamin B6 (mg)	1.6	2.2
Vitamin B12 (mcg)	2.0	2.2
Vitamin C (mg)	60	70
Vitamin D (mcg)	10	10
Vitamin E (mg)	8	10
Vitamin K (mcg)	55	65
Zinc (mg)	12	15

requirement; because you can only have an extra 300 calories a day, make them count by choosing foods that overlap categories.

In addition to what you eat, the way you eat—and the way you gain the weight—is important to you and your baby's health. Frequent small meals help stave off nausea and heartburn, keep blood sugar levels more stable, and avoid starvation *ketosis.* Skipping meals is not healthy, and your mom was right when she said breakfast is the most important meal of the day. Steady weight gain is much healthier than packing on 10 pounds in 2 weeks and then trying to starve yourself the next month to make up for it.

What if you've been indulging in Ben & Jerry's every night up to this point? Relax, you have not done irreparable harm to yourself or your baby, but from now on, let that Chunky Monkey be an occasional treat rather than a routine. A wise saying (who said it I can't remember, probably my mom!) is "All things in moderation." This is true not only for sinful desserts, but also for caffeine, artificial sweeteners, and Big Macs. My rule of thumb for caffeine is no more than two caffeinated beverages a day; ditto for artificial sweeteners or the foods and drinks that contain them. As for high-fat fast foods, sure, on a hectic day it may be all you can get, but drive-thru "cuisine" should be for emergencies and not daily consumption.

Prenatal vitamins are frequently recommended during pregnancy. If you are eating a perfect diet, you really do not need to take additional vitamins, but, let's get real—how many of us are perfect all the time? I like to think of vitamins as an insurance policy; they cannot take the place of a generally well-rounded, healthy diet, but they can help make up for shortcomings when all that stays down is potato chips (my personal first-trimester craving, along with french fries!). Table 11.2 lists recommended daily allowances (RDAs) for women both before and during pregnancy.

Frequently Asked Questions

Q I eat a pretty good diet—lots of fruits, vegetables, and whole grains—but I haven't eaten red meat in years. I do eat fish occasionally, and eggs and other dairy products. Do I have to eat meat in order to get all the nutrients my baby needs?

A *No, you do not have to eat red meat—or any animal products at all—to grow a healthy baby. If you eat fish (a good source of fatty acids for brain development), poultry, and dairy products you will easily meet all of your and your baby's nutritional needs. I, too, have not eaten red meat in years, and I must admit prior to pregnancy my protein intake was not what it should have been. While I was pregnant with Hunter, I was more careful about my protein intake, but that just meant more tuna and salmon and chicken.*

Vegans (strict vegetarians who eat no animal products) do have to be more cognizant of diet. Combinations of vegetable proteins and calcium-rich vegetables, plus the usual fruits, vegetables, and grains will meet most of the daily requirements. Because B12 is primarily found in meats and vitamin D in fortified milk, a good prenatal supplement containing these vitamins, plus B6 and iron, should be taken every day.

Q I cannot function without my cup of Jamaica Blue Mountain coffee in the morning, and I usually drink a 6-pack of diet cola during the day. Do I have to give all this up?

A *No, you do not have to give up all of life's little indulgences, but that 6-pack of cola has got to go. As I mentioned above, one or two caffeinated drinks a day are okay, so keep enjoying that wonderful Jamaica Blue Mountain to get you going in the morning. Sodas are nutritionally empty, plus the caffeine acts as a diuretic (causing you to lose vital fluids), so I recommend good old water as your main beverage. If you need a Diet Coke to maintain your sanity mid-afternoon, go ahead (remember, two caffeinated and two artificial sweeteners a day are okay), but please drink water, diluted fruit juice, or skim milk the rest of the day.*

Q My birthday is tomorrow, and my friends want to take me out for sushi. My mother says I can't eat raw fish when I'm pregnant. Please tell me she's wrong—I love sushi and sashimi!

A *Well, I hate to be the one to break the bad news, but in this case mother knows best! Although the risks are fairly low, there is a* chance of a parasitic infection from eating raw or undercooked fish and seafood. You can still go with your friends, but while they are eating hamachi and maguro, you eat California rolls and unagi.

Another culinary no-no when pregnant is soft cheese like Brie, feta, or Camembert. These may harbor a bacteria called listeria monocytogenes; *listeria has been linked to miscarriages, fetal distress, and stillbirths.*

Week 12

SUN   DATE 11|11

MON   DATE 11|12

↙TUE   DATE 11|6

WED   DATE 11|7

THUR   DATE 11|8

FRI   DATE 11|9

SAT   DATE 11|10

What Happened This Week?

_____

_____

_____

_____

How I Feel Physically and Emotionally

_____

_____

_____

No, You're Not Losing Your Mind, You're Just Pregnant

You WERE EXPECTING the physical changes of pregnancy, but no one warned you about the emotional and mental upheaval. Well, I'm here to tell you that you are not going crazy and you are not experiencing early onset Alzheimer's. Forgetfulness and crying at Hallmark commercials are common, if not commonly talked about, aspects of pregnancy.

What Baby Is Doing

Your baby looks more and more like you every day. The profile is much like you would see on a newborn, with the chin much better defined than it was a few weeks ago. Fingernails begin to develop during this week. All the organ systems have formed; what is left is for them to grow and become functional.

The pancreas begins to secrete insulin and the ovary in a girl is fully formed. Male and female external genitalia begin to differentiate, but it will be a couple more weeks before one is easily distinguished from the other. The portion of the intestines that overflowed into the umbilical cord begins to return to the abdominal cavity. The placenta has taken over the production of progesterone from the corpus luteum.

By the end of this week, the average baby is 61 mm (2.4 in) and weighs 14 gm (0.5 oz.). This is the size of a grade A large egg. The heartbeat should be heard by Doppler in virtually all cases, and on ultrasound the baby is a veritable acrobat.

What You Are Doing

The corpus luteum, that all important progesterone-producing ovarian cyst, is winding down as the baby's placenta takes over that

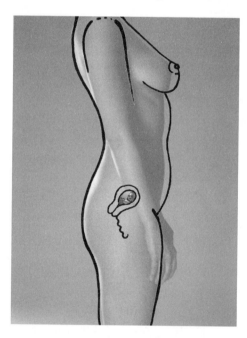

function. Your uterus continues to grow, and now can be felt just at the top of your pubic bone.

You may notice you are broader in the chest—in addition to an increase in cup size, bra size may go up, even before you gain any weight. This is due to relaxation of the muscles and ligaments between your ribs (and everywhere else!) leading to a widening of your ribcage. You may feel warmer as heat production accompanies the 20 percent increase in your basal metabolic rate. My husband delighted in this;

At 12 weeks, you may feel a bit fuller, especially in your breasts, but friends and family will still not be able to tell you are pregnant. Your uterus just reaches the top of your pubic bone.

for the one and only time in our marriage, I didn't complain about his opening the bedroom windows in the middle of a snowstorm!

Special Considerations

You have waited for years to have this baby. Your career is established, you are in a stable relationship, you have gotten used to being an adult. So what's up with the emotional swings? What's up is hormonal chaos, your body being taken over by a little tiny being, and the realization that the comfortable existence you have gotten used to is going to change forever. Even if you already have children, your family dynamics are going to change, and you may be wondering what you have gotten yourself into.

These mixed emotions of elation about being pregnant and fear of motherhood are normal. While these emotions occur in every

From My Journal

(As I was undergoing the infertility treatments, I read *The Language of Fertility*, by Niravi Payne. This is from an exercise in that book.) "'Who says I'm too old?' Well, heck, I did all those years I thought of my parents as old, all those years of telling my mom I wasn't going to be an old fart like her when I had kids. Chronologically I'm older, but in attitude, I'm actually younger. I am not too old—and neither is Jeff—especially not Jeff. He is so young at heart, he's made me younger. Deep down I think I have been afraid we're too old to make such radical changes in our lives—we're so comfortable, but that's just material comfort. What a wonderful challenge it would be to have a baby, to raise a child, to see Jeff changing a diaper! I'm 'younger' and in better shape than I was when I was 20. I am stronger."

pregnant woman, we over-35-year-olds have another, unique unspoken worry: Am I too old for this? Now that I've said it—and I, too, had that same thought many times when I was pregnant with Hunter (and still do!)—you can breathe a sigh of relief. You now know you are not alone. I was 38 when I had my daughter, and although I felt pretty good throughout most of my pregnancy, I worried about having the stamina to raise a child (and I still do!). My mom was 35 when I was born, and I swore I wouldn't be that old and out of touch when I had kids! We are so different than our mothers, though. I am 39 now, but I'm younger than my mom and her friends were at 30; our attitudes and outlooks are not those of the WWII generation.

You can thank those sky-high levels of progesterone in your body for the emotional volatility you are experiencing (and if you haven't cried at a Hallmark commercial yet, don't be smug, because you will!). Being pregnant in many ways is like having **PMS** for 9 months—getting irritated at your husband because he left his socks on the floor, then crying because he didn't notice your new haircut, then smiling from ear to ear as you inform an acquaintance that you are pregnant. You are not crazy; you are pregnant.

Hormones are also responsible for the short-term memory loss that many women suffer. My line when I was pregnant was, "I can't remember anything—all the blood that used to go to my brain is now going to my uterus!" If you go to the grocery store and can't remember what you needed, or if you are in a meeting and draw a blank on your longtime client's name, relax. It's not Alzheimer's, you're just pregnant.

If you have children already, you may be feeling guilty because you are not enthralled by this pregnancy, because you are not keeping a journal to pass on to the baby, because you forget you are even pregnant sometimes. Once again, you are not alone. Just last week, a patient expecting her second child told me, "Sometimes I forget I'm even pregnant, I'm so busy with work and my 2-year-old." You are not a bad mother because you sometimes feel overwhelmed and ambivalent about this pregnancy (and this is true if this is baby number one or number five). You are human, full of joy and doubt and a lot of other messy emotions.

Frequently Asked Questions

Q This is my second marriage, and I have teenagers from my first. I know I'm supposed to be excited about having a baby with my new husband, and we definitely planned it, but we were just 2 years away from having the house to ourselves! Is there something wrong with me that I'm not more excited?

A *The only thing "wrong" with you is that you are a human and not a robot. You have gotten used to one way of life, you've done diaper duty before, and you have experienced the trauma of teenagers. If you didn't have mixed feelings about starting all over again, I'd wonder about you! You are probably also in the midst of first-trimester fatigue and nausea, hardly experiences that contribute to a sense of elation. You do say this is a planned pregnancy, and I bet sooner rather than later you'll be happily poring over baby books and singing lullabies to this baby.*

Q My husband doesn't seem excited about this baby. We planned the pregnancy, and he says he's happy, but he doesn't talk to the baby yet, or rub my tummy or anything.

A *We are all different and show our feelings in different ways. Your husband is probably just as excited as you are about this baby, but he may be having a harder time bonding with something the size of a peach. Many women fall in love with their babies at the moment of conception (if you don't, that's normal too!), but many men need to at least feel the baby move before they experience that deep emotional connection. After one of my first ultrasounds, my husband said he had a hard time thinking a blob of cells was beautiful, but within a few months he was whispering "Goodnight, Hunter" to my belly!*

Week 13

SUN   DATE 11|18

MON   DATE 11| 19

TUE   DATE 11|13

WED   DATE 11|14

THUR   DATE 11|15

FRI   DATE 11|16

SAT   DATE 11|17

What Happened This Week?

How I Feel Physically and Emotionally

Interpretation of Prenatal Blood Tests

ON YOUR FIRST prenatal visit, you had several tubes of blood drawn. No, your doctor is not a vampire; these tests are necessary to ensure the health of you and your baby.

What Baby Is Doing

You and baby have reached the first milestone of your pregnancy: the end of the first trimester. The intestines are now completely within the abdominal cavity; if they remain in the umbilical cord an *omphalocele* results. This hernia of loops of intestines occurs in 1:5,000 births and can be repaired surgically after birth, with little or no long-term consequences to the baby. If the intestines return to the abdominal cavity, and then escape back into the umbilical cord later, this is called an *umbilical hernia*. These are common and often require no intervention, returning to normal by 3 to 5 years of life.

By the end of the third trimester, your baby has grown to 74 mm (3 in) and weighs 30 gm (a tad over 1 oz.). This is the size of a peach slice.

What You Are Doing

As the first trimester draws to a close, you will find that your nausea is abating and your fatigue is not quite so overwhelming. You may have a definite glow to your skin. The increase in metabolic rate and heat generation mentioned in week 12 leads to increased blood flow to the skin as a means of dissipating that extra heat, and hence the proverbial pregnancy glow. Of course, the hormonal upheavals responsible for so many other pregnancy symptoms may leave other women with acne; it certainly seems unfair to be over 35, pregnant, and breaking out like a teenager!

Your uterus can definitely be felt just above the pubic bone, and you may have a sensation of heaviness. Pressure on your bladder, responsible for all those middle-of-the-night trips to the bathroom, should start to ease as your uterus rises out of your pelvis.

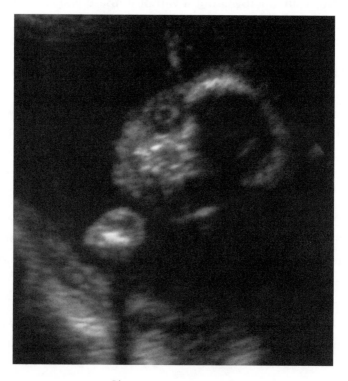

"I've got my eye on you."

Special Considerations

Around the time of your first prenatal visit, you had several blood tests, the standard prenatal panel, as well as a pap smear and cultures. During your second visit, the results of these tests should be available and your doctor will discuss them with you. Often, this discussion only amounts to "All your tests were fine." Well, that's fine, but what do these tests look for? What do they mean?

A typical prenatal panel consists of five blood tests: *CBC* (complete blood count); *RPR,* a test for syphilis; *Rubella* (German measles); *Hepatitis B surface antigen* (HBsAg); and your blood type and Rh status. An HIV test should be offered as well. Table 13.1 lists the typical prenatal panel. African-American women should be screened for sickle cell disease if it was not done during a precon-

---

TABLE 13.1

Interpretation of Prenatal Blood Tests

ABO, Rh

Blood type and determination of Rh status. Incompatibility between the baby's blood type, especially Rh status, and yours can lead to anemia and heart failure in the baby. This is discussed extensively in the text.

CBC

Hemoglobin (Hgb) and hematocrit (HCT). If low, indicates anemia. MCV. If low, may indicate thalassemia, a type of anemia more common in people of Mediterranean or Asian descent. If thalassemia is suspected, additional tests are done.

White blood count (WBC). If significantly elevated, may indicate infection. WBC is usually mildly elevated in pregnancy.

TABLE 6.1

Gonorrhea and chlamydia

Cervical cultures for gonorrhea (GC) and chlamydia, sexually transmitted infections. Both can cause eye infections if the newborn passes through an infected birth canal.

HBsAg

Hepatitis B surface antigen. The majority of babies infected are exposed during delivery. If the HBsAg is positive at any time during pregnancy, the baby should receive Hepatitis B immune globulin and begin the vaccination series within 12 hours of birth.

HIV

Optional but strongly recommended part of the prenatal blood panel. If you are HIV positive, treatment during pregnancy markedly reduces the risks that the baby will become infected.

Pap smear

Samples the cervix and screens for abnormal cells and precancerous and cancerous changes.

RPR

Screens for syphilis. If positive, additional tests are done to confirm. Maternal syphilis can be transmitted to the baby, causing damage to liver, lungs, and bones. Stillbirth may also result. Treatment during pregnancy greatly reduces the risks to the baby if treatment begins early.

Rubella

Tests for immunity to German measles. About 85 percent of people are immune. Primary infection during pregnancy can affect the baby (see week 9, table 9.1). If non-immune, exposure should be avoided and vaccination given after delivery.

ception visit. Tuberculosis screening should be performed in high-risk women (recent immigrants; women in close contact with someone with TB; HIV-positive women; low-income women). Other tests that may be ordered as well, depending on your personal history and risk factors, are glucose screening (obese, history of diabetes with previous pregnancy, or strong family history of diabetes), *CMV* or *toxoplasmosis* (if there is potential exposure), and progesterone levels (if you have had prior miscarriages). Optional testing is displayed in table 13.2.

Blood type and Rh testing deserves a little more explanation, as they can be difficult to understand. We all have two genes for blood type—one from mom and one from dad—and two genes for Rh status. There are three different blood type genes: A, B, and O. A and B are dominant, and O is recessive, meaning you must have two copies of the O gene to be type O. There are four possible blood types, with the genes determining each in parentheses: A (AA, AO); B (BB, BO); AB (AB); or O (OO). The Rh system consists of three *antigens,* the most important of which is D; if a person does not have the D antigen, they are designated "Rh negative;" if they have one or two D antigens, then they are "Rh positive." (Yes, I know this is very confusing!) If an Rh negative woman is carrying an Rh positive baby (because the father passed on a D antigen to the baby), her body may recognize the presence of the D antigen on the baby as foreign, and she may begin to produce anti-D *antibodies.* This antibody production is low in the first pregnancy with a Rh positive baby, but may rapidly increase in a second; these anti-D antibodies attack the baby's red blood cells, leading to anemia and possible heart failure and stillbirth. All of this can be prevented if Rh negative women receive an injection of Rh immune globulin (RhoGam) during each pregnancy; this blocks further production of anti-D antibodies that could attack an unborn baby. If on her routine prenatal panel a woman is found to already have anti-D antibodies circulating in her blood, that pregnancy will be considered high risk and serial antibody levels ("titers") will be drawn throughout the

TABLE 13.2

Interpretation of Other Prenatal Blood Tests

CMV

A blood test to detect cytomegalovirus, a viral infection rampant among children. Most of us, in fact, have been exposed by age 3. Ideally, testing for CMV is done prior to pregnancy in women at risk (teachers, day care workers, and those working in hospital dialysis or infant intensive care nurseries). Those women not previously exposed should be diligent in hand-washing, wearing latex gloves during diaper changes or in the medical setting, and avoiding kissing potentially infected babies and children; these simple precautions markedly decrease the chance of contracting CMV. There is no treatment to prevent or treat a baby infected in utero. (See week 9 for potential effects on the baby.)

"Glucola"

This test, a screen for diabetes, involves drinking a special glucose solution (it tastes like flat, sweet soda) and having blood drawn exactly one hour after finishing the drink. Untreated diabetes in pregnancy has several potential consequences for baby and you. (See week 28 for more information on gestational diabetes.)

PPD

This screen for tuberculosis involves injecting a small amount of the TB antigen into the skin of the arm. If there is active TB, as evidenced by a positive test *and* lesions on a chest x-ray or a positive sputum culture, antibiotic treatment is begun. This decreases the risk of the baby being infected during pregnancy.

TABLE 6.1

Sickle Cell Trait

This screening test for the presence of one gene for sickle cell anemia should be done in all women of African descent; 1:12 African-Americans have sickle cell trait. If positive, the father should be screened as well. If both parents have the trait, there is a 25 percent chance the baby could have sickle cell anemia, which can be detected via CVS or amniocentesis.

Progesterone

As discussed in week 3, adequate levels of progesterone are necessary to sustain the pregnancy until the placenta assumes the role of progesterone factory close to the twelfth week. In women with a prior history of miscarriage, a progesterone level may be drawn, and, if low, supplements given in an attempt to prevent another miscarriage. A low progesterone level may reflect an inherent abnormality in the baby, and adequate levels of progesterone, whether naturally or by supplement, do not prevent all miscarriages.

Toxoplasmosis

This parasitic infection is most often transmitted by inhaling the organism from dried cat feces or eating it in undercooked meat. Most exclusively indoor cats will not have toxoplasmosis. Ideally all cat owners are tested for immunity prior to pregnancy. If you are not immune, give the job of changing the cat litter to someone else. Only a first-time infection during pregnancy will cause any of the problems indicated in week 9. Prenatal diagnosis may be accomplished by amniocentesis and treatment begun; the drug is not sold in this country, but is available through the FDA on a case-by-case basis.

pregnancy. If the titers increase above a predetermined level (usually 1:16), additional testing of amniotic fluid or fetal umbilical cord blood may be recommended to ensure the baby is not becoming anemic; early delivery or fetal blood transfusion is indicated if signs of anemia are present in the baby.

Frequently Asked Questions

Q I had gestational diabetes with my last pregnancy, and there are a lot of family members who have adult-onset diabetes, so my doctor did a test my first visit. It fortunately came back normal. Does this mean I do not have to have the glucola test again at 28 weeks?

A *Sorry, but you do get to drink that lovely glucose drink again! Women at high risk for developing gestational diabetes, especially those who are obese, have a prior history of gestational diabetes, or are Native American, are screened at the first office visit. If that test is normal, screening is repeated at 26–28 weeks. Sometimes the carbohydrate intolerance that marks gestational diabetes is not manifested until late in the second trimester.*

Q I just found out I was Rh negative. I am planning an amniocentesis because I will be 36 when the baby is born. Will being Rh negative affect the amnio results in any way?

A *Being Rh negative will not interfere with the interpretation of the amniocentesis results at all, but you will need to get the RhoGam shot at the time of your amnio. Because the amnio could allow transfer of some of the baby's blood (via placental vessels that are punctured) into your system, this could trigger production of anti-D antibodies. RhoGam is given to block this, even if the placenta is not traversed by the amniocentesis needle, just as insurance. You will also receive another RhoGam injection around 28 weeks and possibly a third after delivery. This last injection will be determined by the baby's Rh status—if the baby is also Rh negative, you will not need post-delivery RhoGam (and, in retrospect, did not need the others, but we won't know the baby's Rh status until after birth!).*

Q I haven't been nauseated for a few days now, after throwing up almost every day for the last 5 to 6 weeks. I had a miscarriage before, and I never felt sick. I'm so worried that not feeling queasy is a sign something is wrong!

A *Disappearance of nausea at this stage of pregnancy usually just means you are entering the wonderful second trimester, a time when many pregnant women feel on top of the world. But you are not alone in your worries: I, too, have had miscarriages, and I, too, was sick as the proverbial dog for weeks and on the day I turned 13 weeks, I woke up and, no nausea. I was so worried I went to my office to listen to the heartbeat! While the lack of nausea is normal, if you are worried, call your doctor's office and ask to come in just for a quick, reassuring listen to your baby's heartbeat.*

Week 14

SUN _____ DATE 11/25

MON _____ DATE 11/26

TUE _____ DATE 11/20

WED _____ DATE 11/21

THUR _____ DATE 11/22

FRI _____ DATE 11/23

SAT _____ DATE 11/24

What Happened This Week?

_____

_____

_____

_____

How I Feel Physically and Emotionally

_____

_____

_____

_____

Telling the World

You are entering the second trimester and have passed the time when miscarriages are most common. If you chose CVS as a means of genetic testing, you have received the results. You will soon be unable to wear your regular clothes. It is time to think about telling bosses, co-workers, family, and friends about your pregnancy.

What Baby Is Doing

Your baby's skeleton, primarily cartilage until this point, begins actually to become bone. The arms reach their final length, relative to the rest of the body, although the legs still lag behind. External genitalia can definitely be characterized as male or female, but not yet by ultrasound examination with any reliability.

An ultrasound at this point will show your baby stretching, yawning, and even sucking her fingers! You cannot feel these movements yet, and won't be able to for another 4 to 6 weeks; it is amazing to watch on the ultrasound this tiny baby doing somersaults that you cannot directly perceive.

At the end of the fourteenth week, your baby is about 8.7 cm (3.5 in) long, the length of a pear, and weighs 45 gm (1.6 oz.).

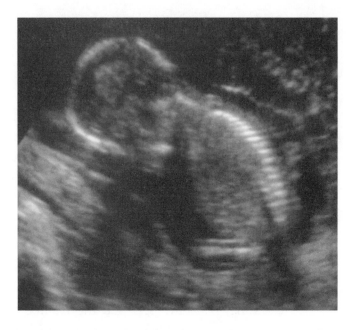

"Sitting down on the job. This 14-to 15-week-baby is sitting down, butt first. The spine is the bright white echos on the right. Five minutes after this frame was captured, this baby flipped completely around!"

What You Are Doing

The second trimester is the "honeymoon" period for many pregnant women. Symptoms like nausea, fatigue, and breast tenderness, which are hallmarks of the first trimester, fade, and typical third-trimester discomforts like swollen feet, backache, and hemorrhoids have yet to appear. Emotional peaks and valleys seem to level out somewhat in this middle trimester as well.

You will probably begin gaining weight at the pound-a-week rate soon, even if you have not noticed any change in the number on the scale yet. Your uterus is two finger breadths above your pubic bone, and your pre-pregnancy pants become impossible to button. Strangers will not have an inkling that you are pregnant yet, but close friends and co-workers may begin to suspect something as your waistline thickens and you take to wearing big shirts untucked.

✎ DOCTOR'S NOTES

After I had Hunter, with the long saga of infertility treatments and miscarriage, I assumed I would not conceive again without the use of fertility drugs (yes, that is dumb, and yes, I know better, but. . . .), so when I found out I was pregnant again, *spontaneously!*, I was both shocked and excited. First I told a few women in my office (my nurse had to draw my blood after all, and our ultrasound tech had to do the ultrasounds). And then, I had to tell one of the general surgeons with whom I was doing surgery—I couldn't just leave the room to throw up without an explanation of why. In any event, by the time I was 8 weeks pregnant, the news had spread. That was when, after two ultrasounds had shown a heartbeat, the next revealed it was gone. I had a D&C that day, on a Thursday afternoon. At 7:15 the next morning I was doing surgery (I could not cancel cases that had been scheduled for weeks and in which the women had made arrangements to be off work); within 15 minutes three people had told me, "I heard you're pregnant: Congratulations!" After explaining to each that I had miscarried, I finally told the third person to tell everyone else because I could not emotionally deal with telling another person the bad news myself.

Special Considerations

Even though you may have called your mom and your best friend the day the home pregnancy test turned positive, you may not yet have shared the news with everyone. Many women, especially those of us who have previously miscarried, prefer to wait to announce their pregnancies until after the first trimester; at this point, the risk of miscarriage is low. Others want to wait until the results of genetic tests are back. It is very difficult to shout your news from the rooftops and then have to deal with well-meaning acquaintances telling you "Congratulations" when you miscarried a month ago.

Certainly, you will want to tell your husband or significant other about your pregnancy right away! Grandparents-to-be and best friends are usually told early on, although who to tell and when is a very individual decision. The conundrum often comes around when to tell your employer, or if you are the boss, when to let your employees know. The best advice I can give is to announce the news at work right around now—before you begin to show. If you wait until you are obviously pregnant, your boss may think you were trying to be deceitful.

As important as when you tell the news is how you tell the news. Tell your boss before you tell the receptionist—that is just good politics. Also, have a clear plan about maternity leave before you make the announcement. Although job discrimination on the basis of pregnancy is illegal, I'd be naïve to pretend it does not exist. If you go to your boss with a statement that you are pregnant and here is the plan for covering your work while you are out; that you will be out X number of weeks, then would like to job share, and here is how that will work, your boss will be impressed and much less likely to assign you only to unimportant work or try to eliminate your position altogether. If you plan to stay home with your baby and not return to work, your employer will need as much notice as possible so you can help train your replacement.

If you are the boss, you should tell your key employees or assistants first. Be sure to let them know you have confidence in their ability to handle things while you are gone, and that you will spend time over the next few months setting up systems to keep everything running smoothly in your absence. Then tell the rest of your employees, perhaps at a group meeting, and reassure them that the business will go on and their jobs are secure. I am in a three-doctor practice, so I took extra calls for several months to help make up for the every-other-night duty my partners would have for the 6–7 weeks I planned to take off. The entire month before I was due, I had a back-up plan in place in case I went into labor when I was on call!

Frequently Asked Questions

Q I am a vice president of a Fortune 500 company and have worked hard at my career, but I want to stay home with my baby. I don't even want to tell the CEO yet, because she didn't quit her career when she had kids. What will everyone think of me?

A *Who cares what anybody else thinks of you—what is important is that you are doing what you think is best for you and your family. And so what if the CEO combined career and family? Some women are not cut out to be home 24/7 with children, and others cannot imagine not being there for every feeding, first step, and temper tantrum. It is the twenty-first century, and we each have the freedom to choose how we want to parent. Stay-at-home moms do not love their kids more than moms who work outside the home, nor do career moms contribute more to society. Raising a family should not be a competitive sport.*

You do, however, need to let your boss know soon about your pregnancy and your plans to step off the corporate ladder, at least for now. You are obviously a highly placed, valuable member of the team, and it will take time to replace you. You can use the rest of your time prior to delivery to tie up loose ends and bring your replacement up to speed. You can then move on to your next career—mommy—with the satisfaction that you did your last job well.

Q Ever since my family and friends learned that I am pregnant, I am getting unsolicited advice about my diet, exercise, even the way I dress!

A *There is something about pregnancy that makes every Tom, Dick, and Harriet think you all of a sudden want their opinions on everything! There is nothing you can do to stop these well-meaning but annoying people from telling you horror stories about their pregnancies or how reaching above your head will cause the cord to wrap around the baby's neck (major myth!), but you can control your reaction to this intrusion. A good approach is to calmly say, "Hmmm, I'll ask my doctor," or "My doctor said swimming is good for me and the baby," or "The story of your 47-hour labor is very interesting I'm sure, but I really want to go into this without any preconceived notions." Polite, but firm, is the key here.*

Q I know I'm not supposed to feel the baby yet, but I swear I feel kicks! What could it be?

A *If you really are only 14 weeks pregnant, what you are feeling is definitely not the baby. One possibility is that you are noticing more intestinal rumblings or gas pains due to the effects of progesterone coupled with the displacement of your intestines by your growing uterus. Another is that you are farther along than you thought you were. A visit to your doctor will let you know if it is possibility number two; if your uterus is much bigger than about 2 cm (the width of two fingers) above your pubic bone, an ultrasound will be done to confirm the age of the baby and your due date.*

Q I had a CVS, and most of my friends know that. We, however, chose not to find out the sex. Everyone I know is pressuring me to find out, because they want to buy the "right" clothes and gifts. I don't know what to do!

A *The choice to find out what you are having before birth is just that—a choice. You have made your choice, and although my choice was different, I admire you for keeping your baby's gender under wraps. It is so exciting at the time of delivery to see whether you have a son or a daughter that it is worth dealing with busybodies now. Tell your friends that white, yellow, green, and purple are always "right" colors, and both boys and girls love rattles and mirrors, teddy bears and mobiles.*

Week 15

SUN   DATE 12/2

MON   DATE 12/3

TUE   DATE 11/27

WED   DATE 11/28

THUR   DATE 11/29

FRI   DATE 11/30

SAT   DATE 12/1

What Happened This Week?

How I Feel Physically and Emotionally

More Blood Tests: The "Triple Screen"

THE FIRST SET of blood tests you had were mandatory, but sometime between 15 and 20 weeks, you will be offered an optional blood test (variously called AFP [*alpha fetoprotein*], AFP-plus, or *triple screen*) to screen for *neural tube defects*, Down syndrome, and Trisomy 18. This test is offered to all pregnant women, not just us over-35-year-olds, but there are additional considerations in our age group.

What Baby Is Doing

During the next several weeks, your baby is growing rapidly. Lacy blood vessels can be seen through the thin, translucent skin. Eyebrows are composed of a few fine hairs, and there is scattered hair on the head and body as well. Tiny hands close to make tiny fists.

The gallbladder is secreting bile, which begins to enter the intestines this week. Bile is what gives baby's first bowel movements their characteristic dark green-black color, but this first bowel movement should not occur until after birth. Bones continue to form, as well as bone marrow. It is highly unlikely that you can feel your baby's gymnastics yet, but he is certainly moving all around his watery home.

Baby is now the size of a mango—10 cm (4.1 in) long—and weighs 78 gm (2.7 oz.).

What You Are Doing

Standing up, you probably still don't look pregnant, but if you lie on your back, there will be a small but noticeable bulge in your

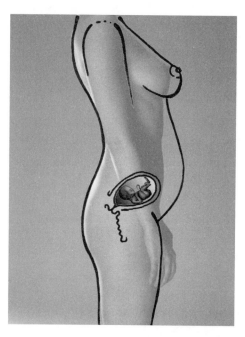

If you started out thin, it is becoming increasingly hard to hide your pregnancy, but if you had a bit more padding, you may not look quite as pregnant as this illustration indicates.

lower abdomen. You may be noticing some heartburn as it takes longer for your stomach to empty and the muscle between the esophagus and stomach is weaker, thanks to our old friend progesterone. Your immune system does not function quite as well as it did pre-pregnancy, so you may catch every cold making the rounds, and it may take longer to shake off minor viral illnesses. You are feeling better than you did in the first trimester, but you still need to take care of yourself—eat a healthy diet, drink plenty of fluids (eight 8-ounce glasses of water a day is the rule of thumb!) and get enough sleep every night.

Special Considerations

Unless you are planning an amniocentesis in the next few weeks (in which case AFP testing is run on the amniotic fluid), your doctor should discuss the triple screen. If you have already had CVS, an AFP blood test should be done, as CVS cannot evaluate for neural tube or abdominal wall defects. AFP and the triple screen are blood tests to screen for neural tube defects and Down syndrome. Neural tube defects include *spina bifida* and *anencephaly,* and result from failure of the neural tube to close properly in the very early stages of pregnancy. Spina bifida means the lower spine has not closed properly; sometimes this is very subtle, with no consequences, but sometimes the vertebrae do not fuse and part of the spinal cord is exposed. This is accompanied by varying degrees of paralysis of the legs and *hydrocephalus,* or "water on the brain." Anencephaly is failure of development of the brain and skull; this is not compatible with life outside the womb.

The triple screen can be drawn between 15 and 21 weeks, but is most accurate between 16 and 18 weeks. The test consists of three components (hence the name!) produced by the baby or the placenta and transferred across the placenta into your bloodstream—AFP; HCG; and unconjugated estriol. All three results are thrown into a formula including your age, weight, and ethnic background, as well as the age of the baby at the time the test is drawn, to derive a number expressed as multiples of a median (MoM) for neural tube defect risk assessment and as an age-based cutoff for Down syndrome risk evaluation.

A result greater than 2.5 MoM occurs in 2.5–5 percent of all women screened and indicates an increased chance that the baby may have a neural tube defect or a defect of the abdominal wall. False positive results can occur if you are farther along than you think, if you are carrying twins, or just as a fluke of the test. If the result is elevated, it can be repeated, as about 30 percent of initially high results will be normal on a second sample. The next step, if the results are still higher than 2.5 MoM, is to do an ultrasound; in almost half of all cases, you will be found to have twins (or more!) or the baby will be older than originally thought. In the remainder of cases (about 1–2 percent of all women tested), a targeted ultrasound is done by a perinatologist. This will identify the vast majority of significant defects, and if none is seen, one can be 95 percent confident that there is no significant neural tube or abdominal wall defect. If no obvious defect is noted, or if ultrasound visualization is less than ideal, an amniocentesis is offered. Once again, the final decision regarding an amniocentesis is up to you; some women are satisfied with 95 percent odds that there is no abnormality, but others want the additional reassurance provided by an amniocentesis. (Week 16 discusses amniocentesis in detail.)

What if the result is low? A low result, expressed as a risk > 1:270, may indicate Down syndrome or other chromosomal abnormalities. In women under the age of 35, triple screen testing identifies about 60 percent of babies with Down syndrome, but in women over 35, the test can detect 85 percent. Amniocentesis is still considered the "gold standard," as is discussed next week, but triple screen blood testing offers an attractive alternative for couples who want some information without undergoing invasive genetic testing. Like an elevated result, a low result may be due to miscalculation of the baby's age, in this case underestimation, or may be due to undiagnosed death of the baby. A low result should never be repeated. An ultrasound is done to confirm gestational age, and if the gestational age is accurate, genetic counseling and possible amniocentesis are recommended.

Like CVS and amniocentesis, the triple screen is a tool to evaluate the status of your baby. It is noninvasive, but it is less accurate than the other tests. Like CVS and amniocentesis, it should be offered to you, but the decision to avail yourself of this test is yours and yours alone. I feel very strongly that all doctors, regardless of their personal beliefs regarding abortion, or their assumptions about their patients' wishes should an abnormality be detected, must discuss and offer the triple screen to all pregnant women, and genetic testing to all women over the age of 35. It is also incumbent upon the doctor to discuss with you the limitations of the test and false positive and false negative rates, so you can make an informed decision whether to have or to decline the testing. In California, where I live and practice, triple screen testing must by law be offered to all pregnant women, and a form signed indicating whether one accepts or declines the test. I also feel strongly that whether or not you choose the triple screen—or CVS or amniocentesis—is up to only you, and no doctor should try to sway you one way or the other.

Frequently Asked Questions

Q I get full so easily—and the heartburn! What can I do?

A *Your stomach does not empty as quickly as it once did, hence you feel full sooner. This contributes to stomach acid, and combined with the sphincter muscle between the esophagus and the stomach relaxing and allowing stomach contents to reflux into the esophagus, leads to heartburn.*

Eating frequent, smaller meals will help prevent that full feeling, and will decrease pressure and minimize the reflux. Avoiding lying down after a meal will decrease reflux and heartburn as well. An over-the-counter antacid, preferably one like Tums that contains calcium (another case of killing two birds with one stone!), can help ease that burning sensation.

Q I'm 15 weeks pregnant now, out of the period when all the organs are forming. Can I safely start having a glass of wine with dinner every night?

A *Just because all the organs have formed does not mean they are not vulnerable to injury. Every system is growing both in size and function. The most rapid period of brain development has not even arrived yet! I certainly would not recommend a nightly ritual of an alcoholic beverage, but at this point an* occasional *drink is unlikely to cause any harm. My rule of thumb, and what I tell my patients, is after the first trimester, a glass of wine or beer on a special occasion is fine, but every day is not a special occasion! If you want to do the safest thing, wait to uncork that wine until after your baby is born.*

Q My husband and I decided not to have CVS or an amnio-centesis even though I'm going to be 41 when the baby is born. I had two miscarriages, and I'm too afraid the testing could cause another one. We are considering the blood test, however. Is this good enough?

A *The triple screen test, plus a targeted ultrasound, can detect 95 percent of cases of spina bifida, all cases of anencephaly, and 85 per-cent of cases of Down syndrome in us over-35-year-olds. There is about a 1–2 percent false positive rate, where the test will come back abnormal even though everything is fine. At age 41, your risk is 1:85, or 1.2 percent, of having a baby with Down syndrome; a normal test result on the triple screen means there is a 0.2 percent chance your baby will have Down syndrome. If these numbers are reassuring to you, then the triple screen is good enough for you.*

Q I am still nauseated every day. I thought it was supposed to go away by now!

A *Hang in there! A few women will have intermittent nausea for the whole 9 months, but the majority will leave the queasiness behind by the end of the first trimester. Studies have shown that only a few women have morning sickness after 17 weeks. Odds are, you will be able to put away those anti-nausea wristbands in a couple more weeks. I threw up almost daily beginning about 6 weeks, but the morning I reached 13 weeks, I felt great. The lack of nausea worried me so much that first day, I went to my office to listen to Hunter's heartbeat to make sure she was okay (obstetricians are the most neurotic pregnant women)!*

Week 16

SUN   DATE 12/9

MON   DATE 12/10

~~TUE~~   DATE 12/11

WED   DATE 12/5

THUR   DATE 12/4

FRI   DATE 12/7

SAT   DATE 12/8

What Happened This Week?

How I Feel Physically and Emotionally

Amniocentesis

IF BECAUSE OF your age-associated risks of having a baby with a chromosomal abnormality, you want genetic testing and you did not have CVS already, you will be scheduled for an amniocentesis right around week 16. Once again, the decision to have genetic testing is yours alone, but I will discuss the ins and outs of amniocentesis in this chapter.

What Baby Is Doing

Baby is rocking and rolling and doing somersaults in you this week—and you still can't feel it! This week, via ultrasound, the eyes can be seen moving back and forth, even though the eyelids are fused. You may even see your baby sucking his fingers or toes, or swatting at the needle during an amniocentesis! It looks like the baby is in the middle of a watery playground.

Your baby will hold her head much more erect now, and the neck is well developed. The eyes face the front (remember they started off on the sides of the head) and the ears are close to their final position. The legs lengthen and are more in proportion to the rest of the body. Unbelievably tiny toenails begin to form.

At 16 weeks, the average baby weighs 110 gms (3.8 oz.), a big increase from just a week ago. Length has also jumped—to 12 cm, or 4.8 in, the size of a small banana.

What You Are Doing

The top of your uterus can be felt halfway between your pubic bone and navel. Because of its size and weight, the uterus can compress the aorta and vena cava if you lie flat on your back. This can make you feel dizzy, can contribute to varicose veins and swelling in your legs, and, of more concern, can compromise blood flow to the placenta and baby. From this point on, you should sleep on your side and should avoid exercises that require you to be flat on your back.

In this second trimester, your blood pressure tends to fall below its normal values. Your heart is working harder to pump more blood to your enlarging breasts, uterus, and the placenta, and the cardiac output will continue to increase throughout this entire middle third of pregnancy. Because of all this extra blood flow, you may notice your gums are swollen, and they may bleed with routine tooth brushing. You may also notice more of a milky vaginal discharge, a consequence of that increased blood flow and hormones.

Special Considerations

You are over 35, and you want to know that your baby does not have Down syndrome or any of the other chromosomal abnormalities that can be detected through genetic testing (go back to week 10, table 10.1 for the incidence of chromosomal abnormalities at your age). You passed on the CVS but have decided on an amniocentesis.

Amniocentesis has been done to detect chromosomal abnormalities for more than twenty years. Amniotic fluid contains cells from the baby, and these cells are grown in a culture medium to increase the amount of chromosomal material available for analysis. Because in most cases the cells from the baby must be cultured, results are not available for two weeks. Sometimes a special technique called FISH (*fluorescent in-situ hybridization*) is used to detect a few specific abnormalities like Down syndrome and *Trisomy 18*; results from a FISH analysis are available in a couple of days. Amniocentesis is usually done between 15 and 18 weeks; earlier than 14 weeks, the risk of complications is unacceptably high, and the practice of early amniocentesis has been abandoned.

The technique for an amniocentesis is relatively simple, but the person doing it must be trained and experienced. Unlike CVS, an amniocentesis may be done by a regular ob-gyn, although some obstetricians refer all their patients to *perinatologists*. Midwives and

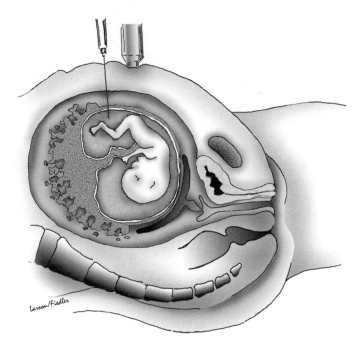

Amniocentesis. Under direct ultrasound guidance, the long, skinny amniocentesis needle is placed into the amniotic fluid, away from the baby.

family practitioners do not perform amniocentesis. First, an ultrasound is performed in order to identify the position of the placenta and the best pocket of fluid. The skin overlying this area is cleansed and, sometimes, anesthetized with lidocaine. Under direct ultrasound guidance, the long, skinny amniocentesis needle is guided into this pocket of fluid; once there, 20–30 ml are withdrawn. The fluid is sent for chromosome analysis and AFP determination. The site of the amniocentesis is watched for bleeding, the baby's heart rate is checked, a Band-Aid is applied, and you are on your way in 20–30 minutes.

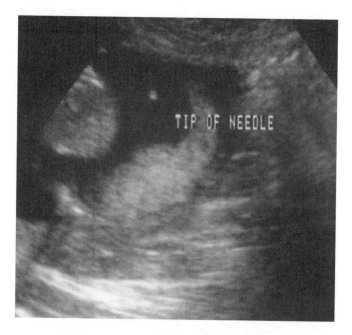

"Amniocentesis. The baby's body is the gray blob on the far left; the placenta is at the bottom. The tip of the amniocentesis needle is the dot. Ultrasounds done during an amniocentesis lower the risk that the baby will be accidentally punctured with the needle."

Like CVS, amniocentesis is not without risks, although the risks of amniocentesis are lower. The risk of a miscarriage as a result of an amniocentesis is 0.5 percent, or 1:200. Other potential complications include bleeding, infection, or trauma to the baby from being stuck with the needle (very uncommon with ultrasound guidance). When doing an amniocentesis, we try to avoid traversing the placenta to minimize risks of bleeding, but sometimes it is unavoidable. Women who are Rh negative will need a shot of RhoGam after having an amniocentesis or CVS (see week 13 for what Rh negative means), regardless of whether the placenta is punctured or not.

TO TEST OR NOT TO TEST

Women—couples—do not take the decision to have, or not have, genetic testing lightly:

Marie S., age 40, having her second child after age 35, did not have any genetic testing: "I knew we wouldn't terminate unless it was something where the baby would die right after birth. I put my faith in God."

Marie B., age 38, first pregnancy, had CVS: "There is a history of Down syndrome on my mother's side. [My husband] told me honestly he couldn't raise a baby with Down syndrome, so we decided to have genetic testing. It was the peace of mind we needed to go forward."

Laura, age 38, first pregnancy: "I had genetic testing—to confront the fears about the increased risk of chromosomal abnormalities and to find out as early as possible if that was going to be a factor in this pregnancy."

Frequently Asked Questions

Q During my amniocentesis, the baby kept kicking the needle. Why did he do this?

A *I'm not sure we can answer why a 16-week baby does something, but your observation is not uncommon. One of the reasons we do an ultrasound is to find a pocket of fluid away from the baby's head or trunk; if we put the needle into a pocket by the feet, for example, and the needle touches the foot, the baby will move it away. We want to avoid touching the baby, but the baby has no such hesitation about touching this strange object entering his space; I often see these little 15–17-week babies grab the amniocentesis needle and then try to bat it away!*

Q I had an amniocentesis yesterday and have been having cramps since. Is that normal?

A *Mild cramping for a day or so after the amnio is not unusual, but anything more than the mildest of twinges should be reported to your doctor. Other symptoms that merit a phone call to the doctor's office are fever, any vaginal bleeding at all, or any passage of fluid or foul-smelling discharge from your vagina. Slight soreness at the site the needle was placed is typical (think discomfort of a shot), but tenderness over your entire uterus is not. If you had previously been feeling the baby move and do not now, report that as well.*

Q My gums are bleeding when I brush my teeth. Is this something to worry about?

A *Bleeding gums in pregnancy are common and are not of the same seriousness that they would be if you were not pregnant. Blood flow to the mouth and gums is increased; the gums become swollen from all the extra fluid in your body, so they are more likely to bleed with brushing or flossing. One in 100 pregnant women gets a benign tumor of the gums because hormones stimulate growth of the tissue.*

Dental care is very important in pregnancy, and you should see your dentist for a cleaning every 6 months. Swelling of the gums increases periodontal disease, and this has been associated with an increased risk of preterm labor and delivery. Proper dental hygiene can help to ward off this complication.

Week 17

SUN	DATE 12/16
MON	DATE 12/17
TUE	DATE 12/11
WED	DATE 12/12
THUR	DATE 12/13
FRI	DATE 12/14
SAT	DATE 12/15

What Happened This Week?

_____
_____
_____
_____

How I Feel Physically and Emotionally

_____
_____
_____
_____

Financial Considerations

H AVING A BABY, raising that child, and sending her off to college is not cheap. Nobody ever seems to talk about the financial aspects of having a baby, but I will in this chapter.

What Baby Is Doing

Your baby's body is covered with *lanugo*, a fine, downy hair. A cheesy white substance (*vernix*) coats the baby's delicate skin to protect it from his watery environment. Vernix is produced by the baby's sebaceous glands and remains quite thick until close to term. *Epidermal ridges* on the palms of the hand and soles of his feet (including fingers and toes) began to appear at 10 weeks and are well established now; these are the basis for our fingerprints, and the pattern they form is genetically determined.

The placenta, absolutely indispensable in bringing vital nutrients and oxygen to the baby and taking waste products away, is about the same size as your baby at this point. It covers a large portion of the uterus at this stage, and on ultrasound it is not unusual to find it covering a portion of the cervix. In the majority of cases, as the uterus expands, the placenta will be drawn away from the cervix; if it does not, a *placenta previa* will result (see week 25).

At the end of the seventeenth week, your baby is 13 cm long (5.2 in) and weighs 155 gm (5.4 oz.). Keeping with our food analogies, this is the size of a cantaloupe wedge.

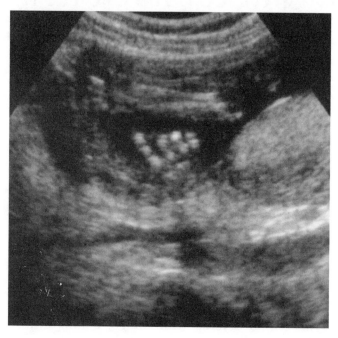

"I'm number one!! The index finger is on the left; the thumb is curled into the palm and cannot be seen in this ultrasound of the hand. All of our babies are number one!"

What You Are Doing

Forget about trying to hide your baby bulge, and go on out and buy some comfortable maternity clothes! Your uterus is the size of a honeydew melon now. The *round ligaments* that run from the upper portion of the uterus to the pelvic side walls begin to stretch as the uterus expands. This can cause an uncomfortable burning or pulling sensation, similar to a "stitch in the side" from running. Because the uterus is rotated toward the left a bit anyway, this stretching sensation is often more pronounced on the right side.

Special Considerations

You and your partner decided to have a baby (or add to the family you already have). You've been taking folic acid, you had a pre-conception visit with your doctor, you have bought a crib and a car seat, and you are taking a childbirth education class (and reading books like this!). You are all set, right? Wrong, if you haven't thought about the monetary aspects of becoming a parent.

The first thing to consider is your insurance coverage. Not all policies automatically cover pregnancy; sometimes an additional premium is required. In other cases, there is an additional maternity deductible in addition to the regular deductible. I found this out when I was pregnant; I knew I had a $1,000 maternity deductible, but what I didn't know was I had to meet that *and* my regular $1,000 deductible before coverage kicked in! The CVS I had at 11 weeks took care of both those deductibles, and after that, everything else was covered. If you do not have insurance, you will have to pay for everything out of pocket, and you must begin budgeting for that now. Speak not only to your doctor for an estimation of her fees, but also to the hospital finance office. Table 17.1 shows average medical costs. Keep in mind that costs vary considerably from region to region; the roughly $2,000 I charge for global prenatal care and delivery at Lake Tahoe is less than half what is charged in New York City!

> *From My Journal*
>
> "You are 17 2/7 weeks and I definitely have a 'baby bulge'—I love my pregnant-looking belly. Not too thrilled about the hips and thighs, but. . . . I'm not sure if I've felt you move or not. It's ironic, for years I've been telling women what to expect and now that it's me, I have no clue! Being pregnant with you is such a wonderful experience!"

You've figured out what prenatal care, labor, and delivery are going to cost. You know what your insurance is going to pay, and you have a good plan, so you are looking at between $500 and $800 out of pocket. You breathe a sigh of relief, because that's not so bad. Don't put the calculator away yet! You will need to buy maternity clothes and new bras, and probably maternity undies, too. If you do not work outside the home, or if you are supplied with a uniform, you can get by with minimal clothing purchases, but if you work in an office or are an executive, then be prepared to hand over that Visa card. Women's feet tend to increase a half-size while pregnant, so you better add some shoes in there, too. See table 17.2 for some of the non-medical costs of pregnancy. And you will need to consider a cut in income while you are out on maternity leave (disabil-

TABLE 17.1

Medical Costs of Having a Baby

Amniocentesis	$900
Anesthesia fee, labor epidural	$725
Anesthesia fee, spinal for cesarean section	$350
Blood work	$300
CVS	$2,200
Insurance premium (1 year)	$2,400
Hospital charges, vaginal delivery, 1-day stay	$4,000
Hospital charges, cesarean section, 3-day stay	$7,000
Obstetrician's fee, vaginal delivery	$2,300
Obstetrician's fee, cesarean section	$2,500
Triple screen	$110
Ultrasound	$350

ity usually pays only a portion of your earnings), and how you will cut expenses if you do not plan to return to work.

You made it through the pregnancy with enough spare change in your pocket to call all the relatives with the good news, but that baby just keeps soiling those diapers—and believe me, those things ain't cheap! I nursed my daughter for a full year, but I had to buy a pump, bottles (and my little princess would only use the Playtex disposable system!), and nipples for when I was at work. And, well, one can get carried away with those cute little clothes! You repeat moms have the advantage that you may have hand-me-downs to use. Film can be another big expenditure, and add in the costs of a digital camera or scanner so you can e-mail pictures to the grandparents. Check out table 17.3 for some of those costs! You will get a lot of gifts, and there is nothing wrong with hand-me-downs or secondhand shops (but always get a new car seat). Even with all that, we spent almost $5,000 on Hunter during her first year of life, plus another $10,000 on one-on-one in-home childcare (and I'm not talking live-in nanny here).

At the same time you are paying for all of this, you still need to

TABLE 17.2	
Non-Medical Costs of Having a Baby	
Bras, underwear, and pantyhose	$100
Manicure and pedicure before delivery	$50
Maternity clothes	$500
Cocoa butter (for stretch marks!)	$25
Shoes (2 pairs)	$100

TABLE 17.3

Baby Stuff, The First Year

Baby food	$500
Bassinet	$150
Bedding and mattress	$250
Bottles and nipples	$150
Bowls, utensils, bibs	$75
Breast pump (electric, double pump)	$250
Car seat	$80
Childcare (day care center, 5 days a week)	$7,500
Childproofing	$75
Crib	$350
Diaper bag	$35
Diaper Genie and refills	$150
Diapers (disposable, bought in bulk)	$1,000
Diaper wipes, diaper ointment	$175
Doorway jumper	$30
First aid and medications	$50
Formula (mix, not ready made)	$1,500
Front carrier	$80
High chair	$60
Layette	$150
Photos (developing, film, portraits)	$600
Stroller (stroller/infant car seat combo)	$180
Swing	$40
Toiletries	$50
Well-baby care and immunizations (co-pay only)	$200

be saving for your retirement and for Junior's college. Right now, the average cost (tuition, room and board, supplies, and personal expenses) for 4 years at a public college or university is $42,000; for a private college or university it is a whopping $90,000! In 20 years, those figures will climb to approximately $137,000 and $279,000, respectively. My daughter should start college in 2016. If she goes to the University of California at Berkeley, it will cost (based on a calculator at *www.usnews.com/usnews/edu/dollars/dscosts.htm?id= 216.162.169.86*) $166,984; and if she attends Bryn Mawr College, my alma mater, it will be a breathtaking $365,175. These numbers do not take into account financial aid of any form, but I still think I'm going to faint!

Frequently Asked Questions

Q Now that I'm starting to show, I'm afraid to wear my seat belt. Won't it hurt the baby?

A *Wearing a seat belt and shoulder harness will not hurt the baby, but forgoing buckling up could grievously harm both of you. No matter how good a driver you are or how short a trip you are taking, you should never put the car in gear unless both lap and shoulder belts are secured. Once you begin to pop out, you should wear your the lap portion of your seat belt under the bulge of your belly, low across your hips and upper thighs. The shoulder belt should rest between your breasts. Worn like this, there is little chance of any injury from the seat belt should you be involved in an accident. If your car has an airbag, push the seat back as far as you can (but not so far you have a hard time reaching the steering wheel or brakes!). The potential for an airbag to save your life is greater than the chance that it would hurt your baby.*

Q My husband and I do not have medical insurance. We do have money saved for the doctor, but I didn't count on how expensive the hospital would be. Do you have any suggestions?

A *Talk to your doctor about discounts for paying cash and about setting up a payment plan—kind of like a layaway. Also, call the hospital's business office; often they will also waive a percentage of charges if you do not have insurance and do not qualify for your state's medical assistance program. Third, don't assume you do not qualify for any assistance: contact the local welfare office for information. Some states have programs to pay for prenatal and newborn care for those women who fall between the cracks: not having insurance provided through their jobs, yet earning too much money to qualify for Medicaid.*

Q This is my second child, after a 10-year break! I look huge already. Am I having twins, or am I going to give birth to a linebacker?

A *While you certainly could be welcoming two into the world (the incidence of twins increases with age; see week 27), it is much more likely that you look so big because of the way you are carrying this baby. With baby number one, especially when you were 10 years younger, your abdominal muscles were tighter. This time around, they have already been stretched out by your first pregnancy and are not able to hold your expanding uterus in so well. Many second- (or more) time moms carry much more forward, which makes them seem bigger. Ignore all the strangers who ask you when you are due and express shock when you give a date more than five months away; if your doctor is not concerned about the size of your uterus, then you should not be either.*

Q At 42, with three kids from a previous marriage, I had pretty bad varicose veins to begin with. I don't want them to get any worse. What can I do?

A *Wearing support hose is the best thing you can do, not only to prevent varicose veins from worsening but also to alleviate the achi-*

ness that accompanies these dilated leg veins. While you may be able to wear your regular support hose now, an investment in a good pair of maternity support hose will provide the best compression of your legs without constricting your expanding belly. Do not lie flat on your back, as this blocks the return of blood from your lower body and increases the pressure in your already dilated veins. Don't cross your legs, for the same reason. Yoga may also help with varicose veins, especially poses where your hips are higher than your heart, like a modified shoulder stand. I used to take a shower, then lie on the floor (tilted to the left, of course, to keep my uterus from putting pressure on the vena cava!), with my legs resting up the wall—I'd pull on support hose this way, so there was no excess blood in my varicose veins.

Week 18

SUN   DATE 12/23

MON   DATE 12/24

TUE   DATE 12/18

WED   DATE 12/19

THUR   DATE 12/20

FRI   DATE 12/21

SAT   DATE 12/22

What Happened This Week?

How I Feel Physically and Emotionally

146

Baby Pictures

Somewhere between 18 and 22 weeks, many doctors do a routine *ultrasound* to assess the baby. Although studies have not shown that such an ultrasound makes a statistically significant difference in population-wide outcomes, many moms-to-be feel better after the ultrasound—and it is fun to see what baby is up to in there!

What Baby Is Doing

Up until now, your baby literally has been skin, bone, and muscle—fat does not begin to be deposited until now. The ovaries in a girl contain all the eggs she will ever have—about 5 million; this will actually decrease to around 2 million by the time she is born.

Facial features are becoming more defined every day. The ears now reach their final position, and stick out from the head—this can be seen on ultrasound, giving a hint of what baby is going to look like. The bones of the inner ear are formed, and your baby can hear sounds transmitted through the amniotic fluid. These sounds are muffled, like ones you would hear while swimming underwater.

Your baby is now 14 cm long (5.6 in) and weighs 200 gm (7 oz.).

Weight increases relatively more than length due to the deposition of fat. Your baby is the size of a baked potato.

What You Are Doing

As you get bigger, you may notice yourself feeling more short of breath. This is due to a combination of a relaxation of smooth muscles in the respiratory tree, increased fluid, and your larger uterus displacing your abdominal contents, which in turn displaces the diaphragm upward. The diaphragm is elevated about 4 cm from its usual position during pregnancy. This mild shortness of breath, for me manifested by an urge to sigh all the time, occurs in all pregnant women and is not by any means a sign you're too old or out of shape for this baby stuff!

Increased blood flow to your kidneys makes these organs larger, and the amount of urine you pass increases by 25 percent. Because the uterus has risen out of your pelvis, and because bladder capacity increases, you are probably not having to go to the bathroom quite as often as you were in the first trimester.

Special Considerations

Here in the United States, the overwhelming majority of pregnant women have at least one ultrasound during their 40 weeks. Being over 35, you may well have more than 1 ultrasound; certainly if you chose CVS or an amniocentesis you had an ultrasound with those tests. If you underwent any infertility treatments, you will have already had an ultrasound to determine how many babies you are carrying.

An ultrasound can be a wonderful tool to assess the health of the baby, but it cannot detect every possible birth defect. A normal ultrasound does not guarantee a perfect child. An ultrasound cannot determine if the baby is mentally retarded, or if he will grow up to have attention deficit disorder. Even when used to clarify your due date, there is a margin of error in ultrasound. The earlier the test is done, the smaller the range of error; an ultrasound done in the first trimester is plus/minus 7 days, while one done in the third trimester has a range of 3 weeks in either direction. This is the reason your due date will not be changed based on a late ultrasound.

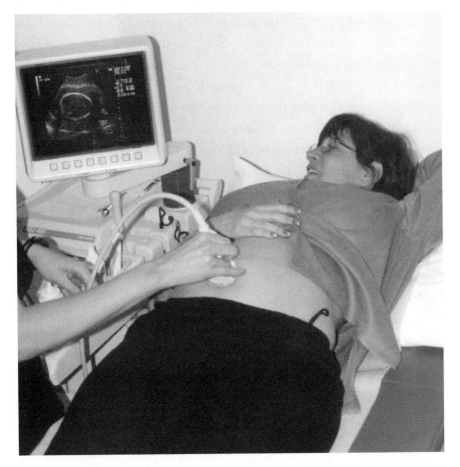

"Better than the movies. Tracy, age 39, gets a good look at her baby's head during a 20-week ultrasound."

Ultrasound is only as good as the people performing and interpreting it, and many studies have shown a higher detection rate of abnormalities in university settings than in either community hospitals or office settings. The basic ultrasound that is performed in many doctors' offices is designed to determine the number of babies, the location of the placenta, the gestational age, and the due date, and to rule out gross abnormalities, but not subtle defects. A *targeted ultrasound* is usually performed by or under the auspices of a perinatologist, and is designed to evaluate possible abnormalities detected on a prior ultrasound or suggested by past history or problems identified during this pregnancy. For example, a routine ultrasound done in your doctor's office should detect anencephaly, where the baby's brain does not develop, but it may not identify a heart defect, where more specialized ultrasound techniques, including color Doppler flow, are necessary. If you have had a child with a birth defect before, your doctor will likely refer you for a targeted ultrasound between 18 and 20 weeks, to see if this baby has the same birth defect. If you have an elevated triple screen test,

✎ DOCTOR'S NOTES

I don't think anyone could possibly have had more ultrasounds than I did when I was pregnant with Hunter (one per week from 5 to 12 weeks [miscarriage fears and CVS], then one at 16 weeks [just because!], then one per week from 19 to 23 weeks [because I though my cervix was shortening], then one per month from 26 to 37 weeks [to check for growth], plus exposure to the same sort of sound waves for fetal monitoring every week from 28 weeks until delivery)—I figure I had about 16 ultrasounds and 12 non-stress tests, and my daughter is perfectly healthy—and brilliant (spoke 100 words in English and Spanish at 18 months!) and beautiful to boot!

which may indicate spina bifida, your doctor will have you get a targeted ultrasound if an early office ultrasound has already confirmed gestational age (being off on your dates can affect the triple screen results, as discussed in week 15).

Ultrasound is a safe test. It works by sending intermittent, high-frequency sound waves from a transducer. These waves bounce off tissues and then back to the transducer, where they are picked up and translated into images on a screen. Theoretically, sound waves can heat up the tissues through which they pass, but with the frequencies used in obstetrical ultrasound, this does not happen. These sound waves have never been shown to cause any harm to a developing baby.

Frequently Asked Questions

Q My nose is so stuffy I can hardly sleep at night. Can I use a nasal decongestant spray?

A *That stuffy nose is yet another manifestation of the increased blood flow and fluid volume of pregnancy. You may also notice postnasal drip or even nosebleeds. All of these symptoms tend to be worse in winter when we heat our houses and the air is drier.*

Try a humidifier (I bought a cool mist ultrasonic humidifier, and after Hunter was born, I moved it into her room), especially in your bedroom. Use saline (saltwater) nose drops freely, but avoid decongestant sprays. The frequent use of decongestant nasal sprays actually causes a rebound swelling of the nasal passages, and you can get into a vicious cycle of congestion, using a spray, and then even more congestion.

Q My neighbor had an ultrasound, which indicated she was going to have a boy. Well, they have a daughter who is wearing an awful lot of blue! How accurate are ultrasounds at determining the sex of the baby?

✎ DOCTOR'S NOTES

Sitting comfortably, tighten the muscles in the vagina and around the rectum, as if you are trying to stop a stream of urine. Hold the muscle contraction for 5–10 seconds, then release. Start with 5–10 repetitions 4 times a day, and work up to 25 reps. You may initially practice Kegel exercises while urinating, again squeezing the vaginal muscles to stop the stream of urine, but once you have gotten the hang of it, do not continue to stop and start urination. You can do Kegel exercises while on the phone, at a stop light, or during television commercials—and no one will be the wiser!

A *I always tell my patients not to paint the room a certain color based on the ultrasound! The ability to determine the baby's gender depends on several factors: the age at which the ultrasound is done; the skill of the person doing the scan; and the position of the baby. Early in the second trimester, the genitalia are not differentiated enough to be able to tell a boy from a girl. By 18–20 weeks, when most routine ultrasounds are performed, one can distinguish sex if the baby cooperates. If the baby is breech and sitting low in the uterus, or if the legs are crossed, or if a loop of the umbilical cord is between the legs, it may be impossible to even see the area of interest. With the right angle, anyone can tell it's a boy, but identifying a girl takes more skill.*

Some radiology departments will not look for the sex. Others will make the effort if you ask, but it is not part of the routine ultrasound anatomic survey. If you do not want to know the sex, be sure to mention that as well so the technician or doctor does not blurt it out.

Q I am not getting up in the middle of the night to urinate anymore, but I am wetting my pants if I laugh or sneeze. I knew

I was too old to be having a baby! Am I going to have to buy two sizes of diapers—newborn and adult?

A *Your age has little to do with your experiencing stress incontinence. Although there is less pressure on your bladder from the uterus at this point, the effects of progesterone on smooth muscle cause a decrease in bladder and urethra muscle tone. This contributes to loss of urine with anything that increases intra-abdominal pressure, like coughing, sneezing, laughing, or exercising. You can do Kegel exercises to help improve pelvic floor muscle tone. Empty your bladder regularly so it does not get overly full. Avoid caffeine (you should be limiting it anyway!) because it is a bladder irritant and a diuretic.*

Week 19

SUN   DATE 12/30

MON   DATE 12/31

TUE   DATE 12/25

WED   DATE 12/26

THUR   DATE 12/27

FRI   DATE 12/28

SAT   DATE 12/29

What Happened This Week?

How I Feel Physically and Emotionally

There's a Whole Lotta Shakin' Going On!

IF YOU HAVEN'T already, you will soon notice the moves and rolls, kicks and punches of the very active little person inside you. If you have had a baby before, you may have already felt movement, but if this is your first, you may have to wait a couple more weeks to feel those first wonderful flutters.

What Baby Is Doing

Your baby's growth slows down a bit compared to that of the last three weeks. *Brown fat,* important in heat production in the new-born, begins to form at the base of the neck, behind the breastbone, and over the kidneys. The lungs are continuing to develop, with formation of respiratory bronchioles and increasing blood flow; the lungs, however, will not be able to function for several more weeks should the baby be born early.

Although the eyelids are still fused, your baby can perceive light and dark. A strong light shone on your belly will produce a warm red glow within the uterus; on ultrasound, babies will turn toward a flashlight held against the mother's abdominal wall.

At 19 weeks, your baby is 15 cm (6 in) long—roughly a medium zucchini—and weighs 260 gm (9.1 oz.).

What You Are Doing

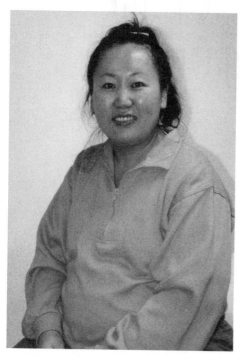

Insuk, 38, has a beautiful pregnancy glow.

Your uterus is just below your belly button, and your profile is definitely pregnant. As you uterus grows, it exerts more pressure on the vena cava, the large vein that returns blood from the lower body to the heart. This contributes to varicose veins—and hemorrhoids. It may also lead to swollen feet at the end of the day, especially in hot weather, or to dizziness if you lie flat on your back. At this point, you should try to elevate your legs when you can, and never remain flat on your back for more than a few minutes at a time.

Special Considerations

Nineteen weeks is when the average first-time mom will feel her baby move. Women who have had a child already are likely to feel the movement earlier, both because they know what to expect and also because the uterine and abdominal muscles are stretched more easily the second (or more) time around. *Quickening* is the old term doctors used to use (and I suppose some still do!) to describe this first perception of movement. The mean time from quickening to delivery is 147 days, $\pm$ 15 days.

Feeling the baby move for the first time is an exciting moment, and for many women, a time of intense bonding with the baby. It somehow becomes much more real when you can feel your baby move inside you. These first movements are often described as "butterflies," but some women do not perceive any movement until the first definitive kick. I will never forget the first time I felt Hunter move. I felt a bit stupid, as patients would ask me if I'd felt the baby move yet, and I'd answer, "I don't know"—after all, I'm the doctor, and I've been telling women for years what these first movements should feel like! When I felt Hunter for the first time, it was unmistakable: it was the day I turned 19 weeks, a Tuesday, and I was driving home from my satellite office in Nevada. I felt a definite "thump," which I knew immediately was a kick. I pulled to the side of the road, tears in my eyes, and called my husband to tell him that our daughter had just said, "Hello."

From My Journal

"7/14/98. I felt you move! Very exciting—this was definitely you, tapping hello. I've felt some weird things before, but wasn't exactly sure, but this time I'm sure—I felt you move!!!!"

Although you now have had the wonderful experience of feeling your baby move—stretch, kick, do somersaults—at this point your perception of these movements is inconsistent. It will be several more weeks before you should expect to feel the baby every day—and before Dad will be able to feel the kicks. There are many factors that influence how well you feel movement. If the placenta is on the front wall of the uterus, it may be more difficult to feel the baby move; imagine someone tapping on your bare shoulder in the summer versus through a heavy winter coat. Ditto if you are significantly overweight. Some babies are more active and stronger than others, too. How busy you are also influences how you feel movement. If you already have children, especially a toddler, you may just be too preoccupied to focus on this baby and its antics. This is something I frequently hear from my patients. When you are concentrating on an important project, you may not notice movements as much. I found this to be true when I was pregnant, not feeling much if I was in the middle of a complicated surgery. The baby is moving, but your mind is focused elsewhere.

Babies have rhythms, times when they are active and times when they sleep. A common observation is that baby is less active when you are more active. When you are moving around, the rocking motion lulls your baby to sleep. When you finally sit down, the rocking stops and baby wakes up. This is a pattern which may persist after birth. My daughter did a full Olympic gymnastics routine every night when I went to bed. Once she was born, if I put her down she woke up and cried. I took to wearing her in a sling and as I went about my business, she would fall asleep. We even bought a vibrating device to attach to her bassinet, which helped her sleep longer at night!

Frequently Asked Questions

Q **This is my first baby and I've felt some flutters, but not the intense, almost painful, kicks my friends describe. Is there something wrong with the baby?**

A *Babies, like those of us already outside the womb, are individuals with unique personalities. Some babies are whirling dervishes, while others are laid-back and mellow. What is important is that you become familiar with your baby's unique personality and pattern of movement. If you notice a significant deviation from what you have come to expect, report it to your doctor. And don't forget, if you are only 19 or 20 weeks, the baby is pretty small—how much punch can you expect a half-pound zucchini to pack! As the baby gets bigger, expect the movements to feel bigger, too.*

Q I've noticed a dark line down the middle of my body, from breastbone to pubic bone. At first I thought it was dirt, but it won't wash off. What is it?

A *This is the linea nigra, a line of increased pigmentation caused by deposition of melanin in your skin. The high levels of estrogen and progesterone in pregnancy stimulate skin cells to produce more pigment. This linea nigra is the result. Some women also notice more pigment on their faces, especially across the cheeks and forehead—the "mask of pregnancy." All this increased pigmentation should fade after delivery. To diminish the chances of an unsightly mask on your face, be sure to wear sunscreen every day and a broad-brimmed hat if you are going to be outside on sunny days.*

Q My husband talks to our baby every night and taps on my uterus to get her attention. He can't feel her move yet, but I swear she kicks him back!

A *You are probably right. Your daughter can hear her daddy, in a muffled, underwater sort of way, and she can perceive light and touch. The more both of you talk to her before birth, the more likely she will be soothed by these voices she recognizes after birth. Unborn babies are curious creatures, and if they notice someone tapping on the walls of their room, they will investigate. If baby is trying to sleep, those kicks back may be her way of telling Daddy to leave her alone—kinda like banging on the floor to get your downstairs neighbor to turn down the stereo!*

Week 20

SUN   DATE 1/6

MON   DATE 1/7

TUE   DATE 1/1

WED   DATE 1/2

THUR   DATE 1/3

FRI   DATE 1/4

SAT   DATE 1/5

What Happened This Week?

How I Feel Physically and Emotionally

Baby Is Exercising— And So Should You

Sometimes all that movement feels as if baby is doing a step aerobics class! That "exercise," if you will, is good for your baby, helping to develop muscles and coordination. Exercise is good for you, too. Being active during pregnancy benefits both mental and physical health, but you may have to make some modifications of your usual pre-pregnancy activities.

What Baby Is Doing

Your baby looks just like a baby at this point—a tiny little person, with hair on her head (although that hair may be pretty darn sparse!), and tiny, perfect fingernails and toenails. Your baby will yawn, suck her thumb, and play with her umbilical cord—little boy babies are often seen playing with their penises, too. In little girl babies, the uterus is fully formed by 20 weeks, but the vagina is still solid.

A 20-week baby weighs 320 gm (11.2 oz.) and is 16 cm (6.4 in) long. This is the size of the salmon steak marinating in my fridge!

What You Are Doing

Congratulations! You have reached the halfway point in your pregnancy—20 weeks down, 20 more to go. You have probably felt your baby move, and if you haven't you will in the next week or two. Your uterus is just at your belly button. After this midpoint of pregnancy, your doctor will begin to measure your uterus; between 20 and 34 weeks, the size of the uterus in centimeters equals the number of weeks, plus or minus 2 cm. A measurement significantly different from this is usually evaluated by another ultrasound.

Special Considerations

The days of considering a pregnant woman a delicate flower, needing coddling and bed rest for the entire 9 months are long gone. Today, I'm more likely to have to tell my patients to slow down a bit. Many of us over-35-year-olds are active and consider exercise an important part of our daily lives, necessary for both physical and mental fitness. Certain activities, like scuba diving, are taboo, and others may need to be modified, but being fit throughout pregnancy can help ward off backaches, constipation, and varicose veins, and it may make labor and delivery a bit easier. Going through labor and pushing out a baby requires as much exertion as running a marathon; you wouldn't dream of running 26.2 miles without training for it, so why would you approach labor any differently? Exercise during pregnancy is training for the marathon of labor.

If you followed an exercise program before you got pregnant, you will need only to modify it as the weeks go by. Pregnancy is not the time to try to set any records for speed, endurance, or strength; moderation is the ruling principle. If you have not been exercising, this is a good time to start—but slowly. First, you will need to discuss your exercise plans with your own doctor. A woman with an incompetent cervix, vaginal bleeding, preterm labor in this or a previous pregnancy, or pre-eclampsia should not exercise.

What are the best exercises or activities during pregnancy? Walking, swimming, and yoga are three that come to mind immediately. Walking at a brisk pace is an aerobic exercise, and aerobic exercises improve circulation (including transport of oxygen and nutrients to your baby), build endurance (very helpful in another 20 weeks

✎ DOCTOR'S NOTES

Before I became pregnant, I lifted weights with a trainer twice a week, for an hour. I also spent about 30 minutes doing some type of aerobic exercise two or three times a week (stationary bike or StairMaster in the gym, or mountain bike, Rollerblades, kayak, or cross-country skis, depending on the season). Being fit was very important to me, and I wanted to continue during my pregnancy. My trainer was one of the first people I told, even before my mother, I think! He modified my regimen to accommodate the pregnancy—after the first trimester, I no longer was supine (flat on my back) for any exercises, I decreased the amount of weight I lifted, and, in the late second trimester, I stopped doing exercises that required tremendous balance (the expanding uterus throws off your center of gravity). I swam once a week, rode the stationary bike (after about 25 weeks, it was too uncomfortable to ride my mountain bike), or walked. When the snow fell, I cross-country skied; I did my last ski run, up a ridge (walking down to avoid falling!), 2 days before I delivered. I also took a prenatal yoga class. Being physically fit from the exercise and mentally calm, thanks to yoga, helped me so much throughout my pregnancy and delivery.

when you go into labor!), tone muscle (a plus in decreasing back-aches and constipation), and burn calories (and you don't want to gain too much weight while pregnant—see week 21 for guidelines on appropriate weight gain). Swimming is also an aerobic exercise. It does not stress the joints, the water keeps you from becoming overheated, and the buoyancy of water can make you feel so grace-ful—a feeling not to be sneezed at when you may feel like a lum-bering walrus on land! Yoga is good for both mind and body. The easy, rhythmic, deep breathing is calming, and a wonderful tool for labor. The stretches and gentle poses appropriate for pregnancy can help prevent backache and varicose veins.

Exercising in pregnancy requires some common sense. As I mentioned before, this is not the time to push yourself to your lim-its. The American College of Obstetricians and Gynecologists has published guidelines for exercise during pregnancy. These pretty closely match what I tell my patients, and what I tried to follow when I was pregnant. The guidelines follow.

GUIDELINES FOR EXERCISE DURING PREGNANCY
(Modified from the American College of Obstetricians and Gynecologists)

1. Pregnant women can continue to exercise using mild to moderate routines. Regular exercise at least 3 times a week is more beneficial than sporadic exercise.

2. Avoid exercising supine (flat on your back) after the first trimester to avoid compressing the great vessels (aorta and vena cava), which may lead to decreased blood flow to the baby as well as to dizziness in you. Avoid standing motionless for long periods of time (this can lead to pooling of blood in your legs, which in turn increases varicose veins and may lead to dizziness because the blood is not going to your brain as well as it should).

3. Modify the intensity of your workout. You should be able to carry on a conversation while exercising. If you are huffing and puffing, you need to slow down! Never exercise to exhaustion.

4. Your changing center of gravity raises the potential for losing your balance. Exercises requiring keen balance may need to be avoided, especially in the third trimester. Contact sports and those involving the potential for abdominal trauma are best avoided as well.

5. Merely being pregnant requires consuming an additional 300 calories per day. If you exercise, you will need to eat additional high-quality foods to compensate for the calories burned during exercise.

6. Avoid becoming overheated at all times during pregnancy, but especially in the first trimester. Drink extra fluids before, during, and after exercise (rule of thumb: 8 ounces of fluid every half-hour). Wear layered clothing that can breathe and wick moisture away from you (synthetics are infinitely superior to cotton in this case), and remove layers as you warm up. If you are indoors, make sure the area is well ventilated, or use a fan to keep the air moving. Avoid exercise in especially hot or humid weather.

Since I live in a mountain community in California, my patient population tends to be more active than the average. A fairly large percentage of my OB patients are over 35, many are having their first child, and many are used to skiing 50+ days a season and hiking all summer. My advice on activities may differ a little from the norm, because of this population, so you should always check with your own doctor and follow her recommendations; after all, she is the one taking care of you and your baby! Table 20.1 lists some specific activities, whether they are okay in pregnancy, and what modifications, if any, need to be made.

TABLE 20.1

Activity Do's and Don'ts

Aerobics Classes

Low-impact classes are okay, but high-impact moves should be avoided. Avoid sudden changes of direction that could cause you to lose your balance or injure your joints (remember, your joints and ligaments are more lax during pregnancy). I recommend avoiding step aerobics because of the possibility of falling.

Bike Riding

On a stationary bike, especially a recumbent one, biking can be done throughout pregnancy. On a road or mountain bike, stick to paved bike paths (no single track, technical mountain biking!). You will probably need to stop biking around the 25–28 week mark as your pumping legs begin to hit your pregnant belly; upright handle bars may let you comfortably ride your bike longer. If you are a novice, please ride only bikes that stay in one place, as biking requires good balance.

Cross-Country Skiing

Excellent winter exercise. Stick to fairly level ground or only mildly rolling hills.

Downhill Skiing

If you are a solid blue or better skier, you can continue, but you must ski one level below what you normally would. No bumps, no trees, no black diamonds, or ungroomed runs. Avoid crowds.

Horseback Riding

If you have a gentle horse you know well, who is not easily spooked, you can ride—at a walk only!

TABLE 20.1

Ice Skating

Similar to *in-line skating*—only if experienced. No jumps or spins.

In-line Skating

Okay to skate on flat, even surfaces if you are very experienced, but no hills and not fast! Do not try if you are not already a good in-line skater.

Kickboxing

The punches of a bag-oriented kickboxing class are fine, and a great upper body workout, but the kicks are a no-no after the first trimester due to the risk of overbalancing and falling.

Running/Jogging

At a slower pace than you usually run, you can continue. No competitive running. Follow the recommended guidelines.

Scuba Diving

Absolutely forbidden at any time during pregnancy.

Snowboarding

Similar to *downhill skiing*. Only the very best of snowboarders should even think about riding during pregnancy—and, like skiers, only on blue or green groomed terrain (in other words, why bother!).

Spinning Classes

Most spinning classes are too intense for pregnancy, but if you do not try to keep up with the instructor and do maintain your ability to talk without gasping, you can spin as long as your pregnant belly does not get in the way.

Swimming

Excellent choice during pregnancy. I don't suggest learning how to swim while pregnant, however!

TABLE 20.1

Tennis

Doubles is best. With singles, there is the risk of joint injury from sudden direction changes.

Walking

Indoors on a treadmill or in the great outdoors, an exercise that everyone can do.

Water Skiing

Nope. Too much risk of injury.

Weight Lifting

If you avoid the supine position and lift lighter than you did pre-pregnancy, weight lifting is an excellent way to tone muscles and build strength. The quarterly magazine *Fit Pregnancy* has an excellent section on weight lifting in pregnancy.

Yoga

Another excellent pregnancy exercise. Try to find a prenatal yoga class, where the moves are gentler and where there is an emphasis on relaxation and visualization.

Frequently Asked Questions

Q I just found out I am pregnant. My husband and I are avid scuba divers and already have booked a trip to the Caymans in 2 months. Can I scuba?

A *No, sorry, you cannot strap tanks to your back and explore the depths of the ocean. The increased pressure decreases the blood flow through the placenta. The compressed air at those pressures does not deliver enough oxygen to the baby. There is the risk of "the bends," nitrogen narcosis, and an embolism. No, you need to stay on the surface of the water.*

You can, however, snorkel. I've been to Grand Cayman and though my husband told me the diving was amazing, I was thrilled to snorkel. The fish are beautiful, and there are some great snorkeling spots a short swim from the beach.

Q I hate to exercise, but I'm already gaining too much weight, so I need to do something. Any suggestions?

A *Even the most dedicated couch potato knows how to walk! I'm not talking hiking up Mount Whitney, I'm talking parking farther away at the grocery store, or making it around the block. Start slow and gradually build up. Walk in the great outdoors and enjoy the beauty of Mother Nature. If you live in a climate unsuitable for walking outside (Florida in July, Montana in January), then make a few rounds of the nearest mall. You will feel better and you'll be less likely to be constipated or have a low backache if you get up and move on a regular basis. You may even have an easier labor—and if that isn't motivation to get off your butt, I don't know what is!*

Q I have been competing in triathlons for years. Do I have to give this up during my pregnancy?

A *I have no problem with you continuing to swim, bike, and run (well, jog) during pregnancy, but I do have a problem with competing and trying to win a race. Exercise is great. Pushing yourself to your limits in order to be number one is not. Follow the guidelines recommended, go out there and enjoy participating in a triathlon, but don't try to break any records. If you can't quench the competitive fires, then don't enter any events—just swim, bike and run for your own enjoyment.*

Week 21

SUN	DATE
MON	DATE
TUE	DATE
WED	DATE
THUR	DATE
FRI	DATE
SAT	DATE

What Happened This Week?

_____

_____

_____

_____

How I Feel Physically and Emotionally

_____

_____

_____

_____

Why Do I Have to Get On That Darn Scale!

I N MY PRACTICE I see the two ends of the spectrum: women who feel it is their right to eat whatever they want and couldn't care less if that means gaining 50 pounds, and women who cringe at the thought of needing to gain over 20 pounds. The proper amount of weight gain is important for your baby's health, as well as yours.

What Baby Is Doing

Your baby's nervous system has developed enough to allow him to swallow amniotic fluid. Most of the liquid is reabsorbed, and the little bit of solid material (mainly shed skin cells) is passed into the large bowel, where it will stay until it becomes part of baby's first bowel movement.

Buds for both deciduous (baby) and permanent teeth are in the gums and may even be seen on ultrasound. If you take the antibiotic tetracycline during pregnancy, it is incorporated into your baby's tooth enamel, causing permanent yellow-brown stains on both baby and permanent teeth.

At 21 weeks, your baby is 17.5 cm (7 in) long—a big banana—and weighs 390 gm (13.7 oz.).

What You Are Doing

As we will discuss in more detail later in the chapter, you should start gaining about a pound a week now. Your uterus is a finger's

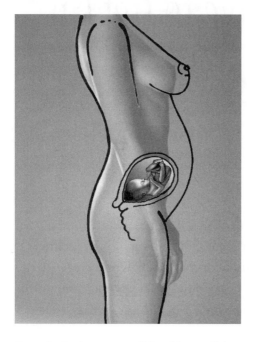

From the back, no one will be able to tell, but at 20 weeks, when you turn sideways, everyone will know you are pregnant.

width above your belly button, and unless you are markedly obese, there's no hiding the fact that you are pregnant.

You may begin to notice stretch marks if you haven't already. Ninety percent of women will get at least a few stretch marks. They seem to be related to both increased *cortisol* and estrogen levels, and are strongly influenced by your skin type and genetics. As your uterus grows—and many women have an almost overnight "popping out" at this stage—*collagen* fibers are torn, and the characteristic reddish, itchy streaks of stretch marks appear.

Special Considerations

Weight. For many American women it is the bane of existence. We are bombarded with images of reed-thin models on the cover of every magazine. We over-35-year-olds have to work harder and harder to keep off excess pounds. Finally, you get pregnant and think you can thumb your nose at the scale, but, no, your doctor tells you you're gaining too much—or not enough. Why do we have to worry about the right amount of weight gain during pregnancy—and what is the "right" amount, anyway?

Excessive weight gain increases the odds of the baby being big, leading to difficulties with delivery; in one study, more than the recommended weight gain was associated with an increase in cesarean section rates from 16 percent to 22 percent. Excess weight leads to more backaches and varicose veins and hemorrhoids and fatigue. You are more likely to develop gestational diabetes or high blood pressure, conditions that you are more likely to develop

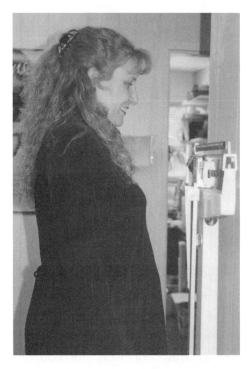

Diana, age 35, is pleased—her weight gain is right on target.

anyway due to age alone; gaining too much weight just increases the chances.

Inadequate weight gain has its own set of problems, such as prematurity and low birthweight. Low-birthweight babies are more likely to develop high blood pressure, heart disease, and strokes as adults. If you don't gain enough weight, you may not be supplying all the nutrients your baby needs—or that you need. Your baby will take iron and calcium from you, increasing your own anemia and fatigue, and possibly increasing the chances of osteoporosis later in life.

In the first 8–10 weeks, the goal is only to gain a pound or two, but due to morning sickness, you may actually lose a couple of pounds. From then to about 20 weeks, you should gain another few pounds for a total weight gain at the halfway point of roughly 6–10 pounds. From 20 weeks on, a pound a week is the rule of thumb,

TABLE 21.1

Where Does That Weight Go?

Baby	7.5 lb. (3400 gm)
Amniotic fluid	1.75 lb. (800 gm)
Blood	2.75 lb. (1450 gm)
Breasts	1 lb. (405 gm)
Fat stores	7 lb. (3345 gm)
Fluid retention	3 lb. (1480 gm)
Placenta	1.5 lb. (650 gm)
Uterus	2 lb. (970 gm)

although in the last couple of weeks, you may not have much of an appetite and may not add any weight. For a woman of average height and pre-pregnancy weight, total weight gain should be 25–35 pounds. (See table 21.1 for where that weight goes.) If you are carrying twins, aim for about 40 pounds. If you were underweight to start off, your weight gain should be at the higher end of the range, or a bit beyond, but if you were significantly overweight, you will be asked to limit your weight gain to about 18 pounds. Even if obese, you should not go on a restrictive diet when pregnant, as the baby will not be able to get all the nutrients he needs.

Frequently Asked Questions

Q My mother, who looks upon my pregnancy as the 9 months she is allowed to give me advice, tells me I'm eating too much. She says that when she was pregnant with me, 36 years ago, her doctor told her to gain no more than 15 pounds. Why have things changed so much?

✎ DOCTOR'S NOTES

I have a small confession here. I may be an obstetrician, and I may know exactly what a pregnant woman should do, but that does not mean I always follow my own advice. I am human, with faults, just like you. When I was pregnant with my daughter, I ate better than I have in my entire life. But in college I was anorexic; 15 years later when I was pregnant, the thought of gaining 25–35 pounds freaked me out. I only gained 18 pounds during my pregnancy and ultrasounds indicated that Hunter was growing well, but when she was born at 39 weeks, she weighed 5 lb. 13 oz., just 5 ounces above the definition of low birthweight. I felt guilty. "I starved my baby!" was all I could think. At 18 months of age (her last well-baby check-up), she was 27 pounds and 33 inches tall (about the eightieth percentile for both), beautiful, active, and incredibly smart, but if I had it to do over again, I'd try to gain closer to the recommended 25 pounds!

A *We no longer confine women to bed for a week after a vaginal delivery, either! Thirty-nine years ago, when my mom had me (at age 35, which in 1960 was old to be having one's first child), she smoked a pack of cigarettes a day, had her cocktail with dinner, and probably only gained 15 pounds, too. I joke and tell her that I'd have won a Nobel Prize by now if she hadn't done all those things! We are much more aware now of the importance of good nutrition and weight gain—not too little, not too much—in growing the healthiest babies possible.*

Medicine is an evolving art and science, and I suspect that when my daughter pulls this book off the shelf 30 years from now, she'll be amazed that in the year 2000 we were so barbaric as to stick a needle in the amniotic fluid to test for genetic defects. By the time our children are having their children, there will probably be completely noninvasive ways to assess the health of unborn babies.

Q I just got back from the doctor's and I think the scale must be broken—it said I've gained 10 pounds in the past month, and 25 so far this pregnancy—and I'm only halfway there! I'm not eating any more than usual, except I have such a craving for chocolate. What am I going to do?

A *That extra weight is history. What you have to do is toss the candy bars and brownies and start eating better—now. You should not try to diet to make up for the excess weight you have already gained; baby needs his nutrients and he needs them all the time. A crash diet now could produce a growth-restricted baby later. If you eat the recommended amounts of the foods in week 11, table 11.1, and if you exercise moderately, you'll be able to gain the small and steady amount each week that is necessary to grow a healthy baby.*

Q I didn't have any stretch marks with my 8-year-old daughter, but this time . . . ! I am having twins, and I know I'm bigger—and older, but this is ridiculous. Is there anything I can do to prevent any more of these ugly stretch marks?

A *It is inevitable that you are going to be bigger and your skin stretched more tautly because you are carrying twins. Being older, your collagen is probably not what it was when you were 18, or even 25. The result: stretch marks. Despite all the claims of the cocoa butter manufacturers, there are no creams or magic potions to prevent these badges of motherhood, although I faithfully slathered Palmer's Cocoa Butter on my belly twice a day (actually, I didn't get any stretch marks but that has more to do with genes than creams). After deliv-*

ery, the wide, red marks you have now will fade to wavy, silvery lines, reminding you that you have done a most wondrous thing—given birth. If you look on stretch marks as a badge of honor, a wise woman said to me once, they no longer seem so ugly. If, after the babies are born, you still hate the way they look, see a dermatologist; vitamin E oil (which you can use in pregnancy), Retin A (which you should not use until after the babies are out), or laser may help remove the stretch marks.

Week 22

SUN _____ DATE _____

MON _____ DATE _____

TUE _____ DATE _____

WED _____ DATE _____

THUR _____ DATE _____

FRI _____ DATE _____

SAT _____ DATE _____

What Happened This Week?

_____

_____

_____

How I Feel Physically and Emotionally

_____

_____

_____

_____

Baby, Oh Baby, the Places You'll Go

MANY OF US like to travel for vacations or to visit far-flung family. Some of us have to travel for business. Traveling during pregnancy is certainly doable, and can be enjoyable, with a few precautions and caveats.

What Baby Is Doing

If your baby is a boy, this week his testes will begin their slow descent from their current position near the kidneys. Your little girl has as many eggs as she ever will; in fact, she will lose millions between now and birth.

Hair on the head is continuing to grow, and eyebrows are more defined. Melanin, the pigment that determines hair color, will not be present for a few more weeks, however. Sometimes, especially with Latino or African-American babies, hair may be seen floating around the head like a halo, even this early!

Your baby is 19 cm long (7.6 in) and weighs 460 gm (16.1 oz.—a pound!)—about the length of a carrot (at least the ones in my fridge), but a lot heavier.

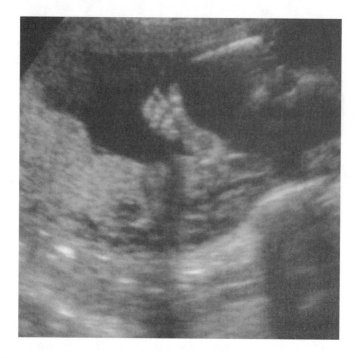

"These feet were made for walking—but not for another year or more! Five perfect toes are on a tiny foot."

What You Are Doing

Every week you get bigger and bigger. Your uterus is now 2 finger widths above your belly button, and if you see your doctor this week, she will measure your uterus with a measuring tape; from the top of the pubic bone to the top of your uterus should be 22 cm ± 2 cm. You are probably feeling the baby more consistently now, and may be able to determine your baby's particular patterns of activity and sleep.

Your sleep may be disturbed by baby's acrobatics at night, or by *restless leg*. This is characterized by a twitching and a burning sensation in one or both calves, with a feeling like you absolutely *must* move around. Affecting 10–15 percent of pregnant women, this usually hits 15 minutes or so after going to sleep.

Special Considerations

We are a nation that likes to get in our cars (or on buses or airplanes) and go. This is the best trimester in which to travel, beyond the first trimester with its nausea, fatigue, and risk of miscarriage, and before the third trimester with swollen feet, backaches, and labor on the horizon. If you are having your first baby, this is a great opportunity for you and your mate to get away for one last time alone (and without having to schlep an inordinate amount of stuff for a small person!). If you already have children, you may want to farm them out so you two can have some much-needed adult time before your newest family member arrives.

Before you book any trips, be they for pleasure or for business, be sure to check with your

From My Journal

"8/3/98 (22 weeks). I feel you move every day now. If I haven't felt you in several hours, I ask you to give me a little tap, and you usually do—thank you for reassuring your neurotic mother! . . . I wonder when Jeff will be able to feel you move? He'll love that. He loves you and worries about you, too. He probably worries more about *me* worrying, though!"

doctor. If you have had any complications with this pregnancy, or have a history of preterm labor with a prior one, travel may be out of the question. Also, you may have to think twice about where you travel while you are pregnant. White water rafting is not a good idea, nor is hiking in the Himalayas. Travel to high altitudes, especially over 10,000 feet, can increase the risk of preterm labor or rupture of the membranes. Also, at these high altitudes, oxygen content is lower; for you this may mean shortness of breath, but for baby it could lead to fetal distress. Be careful about trips to developing countries as well. In some cases, you may not be able to get vaccinated for diseases that are endemic to that area (yellow fever is one vaccine that should not be given to pregnant women). If you must travel to a country requiring vaccines, contact the Centers for Disease Control and Prevention Travelers' Health Hotline at 877-FYI-TRIP (or check out the Web site at http://www.cdc.gov/travel/pregnant.htm) for information on what is absolutely necessary and safe to use during pregnancy. If you do go to a developing country, drink bottled water and avoid eating raw, unpeeled fruits and vegetables. Afraid of dehydration that would accompany a case of *tourista*, we postponed our annual trip to Mexico until after I delivered—Hunter was drinking salsa-flavored breast milk in Puerto Vallarta when she was 10 weeks old, though!

> ## ✎ DOCTOR'S NOTES
>
> Being over 35, many of us don't have healthy, vigorous parents who can help out with this new baby or take other grandchildren for the weekend, especially if, like mine, your parents were over 35 when they had you. Don't let this stop you from getting away, however. Enlist siblings or close friends or a trusted baby-sitter so you can take at least a weekend for yourself before this new baby arrives.

If you do travel, use common sense, too. Don't try to pack too much into a day; you are pregnant and you do need extra rest. Don't try to pack too much into your suitcase either; you don't want to ruin your vacation because you strained your back trying to hoist a heavy bag. Continue to eat as healthily as you would at home. Drink plenty of water (bottled if you are in a foreign country!) so you do not become dehydrated—this is especially important if you are somewhere hot or high.

If you are flying, book an aisle seat. Get up and walk every 30 minutes or so (once the seat belt sign has been turned off!), drink lots of water (the recirculated air on planes is very dehydrating), and empty your bladder several times, including before landing, in case there is a long wait to get to the gate. In addition to walking frequently to avoid swelling and the much more dangerous blood clots in the legs, wear maternity support hose while flying. Elevate your legs, if possible, while you are seated. If you are traveling by bus or car, do the same things (obviously, you can't walk around in a car, but you can stop every 45 minutes to an hour so you can get out and stretch your legs). Always, always, always wear your seat belt in a car (and plane and bus if available)! Taking a cruise can be a wonderfully relaxing vacation for a pregnant woman, and today's huge cruise ships have stabilizers that minimize the rolling motion that plagued those plying the seven seas in the past. Bring accupressure bands along, just in case seasickness hits anyway.

In the last month of pregnancy, it is not a good idea to go too far from home; you don't want to be delivered by a strange doctor in a strange hospital in a strange town, do you? Domestic airlines tend to prohibit flying after 36 weeks, and international ones after 32 weeks. You can get a note from your doctor stating how many weeks you are to avoid hassles at the gate. After about 28 weeks, I like to see my patients before they leave on a long trip; this way I can assess whether there is anything amiss that may preclude travel.

Frequently Asked Questions

Q I am in the middle of the second trimester and doing great so far, but with my last pregnancy I went into preterm labor at 29 weeks. I have an important sales meeting in a few weeks, at Lake Tahoe, which is only a four-hour drive away. Can I go?

A *Unless you want to meet me in person, be placed on drugs to stop your contractions, and maybe take an ambulance ride to the nearest hospital with an intensive care nursery if your labor cannot be stopped,* please *do not go to Tahoe—or Vail or Aspen or any place else higher than 4,000–5,000 feet! The combination of dry air (and result-ant dehydration) and lower oxygen availability increases the chance of preterm labor in someone who is already at risk, based on your his-tory. I can't cite a lot of scientific studies on this, but I sure can tell you I've been up many, many times in the middle of the night getting an ambulance or a helicopter up to Tahoe to take away someone just like you!*

Q My husband wants to take me away for a romantic week-end before the baby is born. He's planned dinner at a fancy restaurant and a stay at a spa. It sounds like fun, but I can't drink and I can't go in the sauna, so I'm feeling like it is a waste of money that we could use for the baby.

A *Believe me, you will be making sacrifices galore once this baby is born—you don't need to start now! You may not be able to share a bottle of an '82 Bordeaux with your husband, but you can enjoy the food. You may not be able to go into the sauna, but you can get a mas-sage and a facial. When I was 16 weeks pregnant I traveled to New York City on business, and my husband joined me after a couple of days. We had dinner at Le Cirque 2000, an incredible visual and gus-tatory experience—I couldn't have the wine, but I sure did enjoy the chef's tasting menu, a decadent dessert (and ate extra healthy the rest of the week to make up for it!), and the impeccable service. Go on this weekend with your husband before you start calling yourselves Mommy and Daddy; after all, how often does a guy suggest something like this—take advantage of it!*

Q I have restless leg and it's making me crazy! Those cramps in the middle of the night are so painful! How can I prevent it and what do I do if it does happen?

A *The twitches and spasms of restless leg can be quite uncom-fortable, not to mention detrimental to a good night's rest. Although* not scientifically proven, restless leg seems to be related to calcium and perhaps magnesium deficiency. If you are only taking a prenatal vitamin, add a calcium/magnesium supplement. In case potassium deficiency plays a role, be sure to eat potassium-rich foods like raisins and bananas regularly.

Stretching your calves before retiring for the evening may prevent the spasms as well. One easy stretch is to stand about 3 feet from a wall, step one foot forward and then lean into the wall, stretching the other calf. To stretch the bottoms of your feet, roll them over a bottle. If you do get a spasm in the night, straighten out your leg and then pull your toes upward; do not point your toes, as this will make the cramp even worse!

Week 23

SUN _____ DATE _____

MON _____ DATE _____

TUE _____ DATE _____

WED _____ DATE _____

THUR _____ DATE _____

FRI _____ DATE _____

SAT _____ DATE _____

What Happened This Week?

_____

_____

_____

_____

How I Feel Physically and Emotionally

_____

_____

_____

_____

Mirror, Mirror on the Wall

You are over 35 and pregnant. Do you feel like a sexy fertility goddess or like an old beached whale? Pregnancy can be a time of incredible sexuality—and a time when your body image takes a beating.

What Baby Is Doing

The last 4-week stretch was one of relatively slow growth, but this week marks the beginning of a time of substantial weight gain. *Rapid eye movements* (REM), like you have when dreaming, begin this week and can be seen on ultrasound. You may wonder what in the world your 23-week baby could possibly be dreaming about—probably just like us, they dream about things they have been doing, like playing with the umbilical cord or the sensation of sunlight shining on your pregnant belly on a warm summer's day. REM sleep encourages brain development, and is, therefore, an important part of your baby's time in the womb.

An average 23-week baby is 20 cm (8 in) long and weighs 545 gm (19 oz.). This is (according to the contents of my refrigerator) the size of a shucked ear of sweet summer corn!

What You Are Doing

Your breasts continue to enlarge. By this twenty-third week, they are almost a half-pound heavier than they were before you conceived. The areola is bigger in diameter and darker, and you may be able to express a small amount of *colostrum* if you massage your breasts and nipples. Nipple stimulation may also cause your uterus to contract, so don't keep massaging those puppies just to see milk leak out! You may notice some stretch marks on your enlarging breasts as well as on your belly.

Because your expanding uterus puts pressure on the ureters as they cross the bony pelvic brim, the ureters and the kidneys may become slightly dilated at this point. This mild degree of *hydro-*

DO YOU SEE WHAT I SEE?

I thought I looked great when I was pregnant, maybe because I had been trying for years to get there and I rejoiced in the bulging belly. Many of my patients, when asked about the worst thing about being pregnant, referred to the way they looked.

Marie, age 38: "I discovered I have obsessed over my weight all my life. It continued into pregnancy. One month I gained 11 pounds. I was depressed for days over that. Pregnancy was very hard on my self image."

Laura, age 38: "Being sick, tired, the body changes that are out of my control—feeling fat."

Kim, 40, and about to have her second by repeat cesarean section: "I'm just so tired all the time. . . ."

nephrosis, or dilation of the kidneys, is normal in pregnancy.

Special Considerations

Your self-image will go through changes as enormous as the ones in your body. Many pregnant women complain in public about the weight gain and the soft, round curves of pregnancy, but in private may revel in their new bodies. Many dads-to-be are incredibly turned on by this full, fertile shape as well. We seem to be afraid to talk about our sexuality when we are pregnant, perhaps thinking that sexual feelings and thoughts are inappropriate for mothers—part of the whole Madonna (the Virgin Mother, not the singer!) image. Well, ladies, I'm here to say you are sexy, your husbands think you're sexy, and it is more than okay for you to think you're sexy, too!

Many pregnant women report they want and enjoy sex more during pregnancy. Others note a definite drop in desire. The bottom line is that preg-

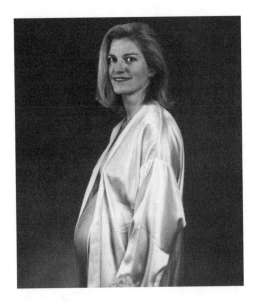

"Me, at 29 weeks. I may not be Demi Moore, but I think I looked better pregnant than I have my entire life."

✎ DOCTOR'S NOTES

I have always had some body image problems—I don't like my chin, I have fat thighs, my butt is too big, and so on. I can honestly say I felt beautiful when I was pregnant. I glowed. My husband thought I was gorgeous. I was one hot mama-to-be and I have the Demi Moore–style photos to prove it!

nancy, if you haven't figured this out already, is a time of change. And things can change from week to week in the same woman! A bit more than half of the women in one survey reported a decrease in sexual desire in the first trimester; well, no kidding—you were too busy throwing up to want to have sex and have someone touch those tender breasts! In the third trimester, it may wane again as the mere logistics of sex (that belly does get pretty big) become more challenging. But this second trimester is often a time of heightened libido. The increase in blood flow to the vulva, vagina, and clitoris can enhance sensitivity and may increase orgasms. Your breasts are not quite as tender, but they are still sensitive, and let's not forget we live in a society where the ideal sexual woman has large breasts and you definitely could be a Victoria's Secret bra model now!

Some parents-to-be worry that sex will harm the baby; in fact, the man usually has this fear. We over-35-year-olds may have had to work hard to get pregnant, undergoing fertility treatments or having had miscarriages in the past, and these fears may be greater than for couples who have never had such challenges. With few exceptions (see table 23.1), sex is perfectly safe and will not harm the baby. This doesn't mean baby won't notice anything; with orgasm your uterus may contract, and in one very interesting study done in Scandinavia, monitoring dur-

From My Journal

"My trainer said the other day that I act like I'm the first and only woman who's ever been pregnant. It's true—I am amazed and enthralled by this pregnancy. I love the big belly, the full breasts, I adore the feeling of you moving, the knowledge that from the love Jeff and I share, a new person—you—has been created. It is a miracle and I rejoice in it. I may be a doctor, an ob-gyn no less, but this is not science and physiology, this is art, this is magic."

ing intercourse revealed the baby's heartbeat increased when either parent had an orgasm.

Whether you couldn't care less about sex during your pregnancy or your sheets are smoking, it is important that you realize your feelings are normal. It is also important for you and your partner to communicate with each other. If he is afraid to make love to you for fear of hurting the baby, but you think he's avoiding sex because he thinks you are unattractive, this miscommunication only makes

TABLE 23.1

When Sex Is Taboo

1. **Bleeding in the first trimester.** Although this frequently is from a mild infection or tearing of the engorged blood vessels of the cervix, avoid sex until you have seen your doctor and gotten the okay to resume.

2. **Placenta previa.** The placenta covers the cervical opening, and sex may lead to bleeding caused by the penis impacting on the cervix. (Placenta previa is discussed in detail in week 25.)

3. **Incompetent cervix and/or placement of a cerclage.** If the cervix is unusually weak and prone to open without labor, a stitch (cerclage) may be put in place at around 14 weeks to keep the cervix closed. Sex (and orgasm) are taboo because they could precipitate contractions.

4. **Preterm labor.** As with an incompetent cervix, orgasm could lead to contractions. Semen itself may also contain substances that could provoke labor.

5. **Rupture of the membranes.** If the "water bag" that your baby lives in has ruptured, sex could introduce infection.

both of you frustrated. And if the tables are turned, and you just don't feel like having sex but are "going along with it," you may feel resentful. If you communicate, as a couple you can find ways of expressing your love for one another that are mutually pleasing. Compromise, as you will be forced to learn once the baby is born, is not defeat, but rather a way of ensuring happiness for all.

If your doctor has made sex off-limits due to any of the conditions in table 23.1, this does not preclude all intimacy. What is forbidden is vaginal penetration and orgasm for you. Unless your membranes are ruptured, oral sex on you may be okay (but not to the point of orgasm), and you certainly can perform oral sex on your mate; always ask your doctor specifically about what can and cannot be done. Cuddling and closeness are always okay and, even if there are no conditions that prevent you from having sex, may be all you want in the first place.

Frequently Asked Questions

Q I have an incompetent cervix and had a cerclage placed at 14 weeks. The instructions said "pelvic rest." What exactly does that mean?

A Pelvic rest *is a genteel way of saying nothing in your vagina— no tampons, no douches, no penises, no fingers, nothing at all. It also usually implies avoidance of orgasm, which might precipitate contractions. Stimulation of your clitoris either manually or orally is okay, but not to the point of orgasm. Anal penetration is okay as well, as long as this is something with which you are comfortable (many women do not willingly engage in anal penetration, and you should never do something you personally find distasteful or painful).*

Usually after the cerclage is removed at 37 weeks, your doctor will give you the go-ahead to resume intercourse. Of course, then you may have to be creative in finding positions to accommodate your belly!

Q I had always heard oral sex was off-limits in pregnancy, but you said it is okay. What gives?

A *Oral sex performed on you* (cunnilingus) *is safe as long as your partner is careful not to blow air into your vagina. The extra-dilated blood vessels in the vagina during pregnancy increase the risks of an air embolism—when an air bubble has traveled through your blood stream and lodged in the lungs. This can be quite serious, because it interferes with oxygenation of your blood.*

Your partner may not be as interested in performing oral sex on you during pregnancy due to the increase in vaginal discharge that occurs. Your taste and smell may be different. Some find this erotic, but others are turned off. Once again, good communication is key, so no one feels rejected.

Q My husband is 50 and I am 42. Our sex life was not terribly active before pregnancy, but now it is nonexistent. I'm not interested and he has a difficult time maintaining an erection. I'm afraid he doesn't find me attractive.

A *Attraction may have nothing to do with it. Your husband may have the desire, but fears of hurting the baby or worries about raising and providing for a child may be in the back of his mind all the time, interfering with performance. He may be unnerved by the mere math of having a child at his age ("When she's 18, I'll be 68."). He may worry that sex is uncomfortable for you. He may not have any of these concerns, but may find it more difficult to maintain an erection because you feel different—moister due to increased secretions and fuller due to engorgement of vaginal tissues with all that extra blood.*

Again, I cannot emphasize how important it is to communicate. You said you don't have much desire—maybe you both would be fulfilled with kissing and caressing and telling each other how much you love one another and this baby you have created.

Week 24

SUN _____ DATE _____

MON _____ DATE _____

TUE _____ DATE _____

WED _____ DATE _____

THUR _____ DATE _____

FRI _____ DATE _____

SAT _____ DATE _____

What Happened This Week?

_____

_____

_____

_____

How I Feel Physically and Emotionally

_____

_____

_____

_____

Born Too Soon

T HIS WEEK MARKS the earliest your baby could possibly survive with intensive, high-tech care if born prematurely. Survival rates increase and long-term complication rates decrease the closer the baby gets to his due date.

What Baby Is Doing

This twenty-fourth week is the beginning of *viability,* or the ability to survive on his own should your baby be born now. Up until now, the lungs could not function, but at this point terminal sacs form in the lung, with blood-bearing capillaries separated by the thinnest of membranes from the (once birth occurs) air-filled *alveoli.* Before this, oxygen in the lungs could not get into the circulatory system. Also, *surfactant* begins to be produced in small amounts; surfactant production will increase dramatically in the last few weeks of pregnancy. Surfactant forms a film over the walls of the terminal sacs, allowing them to remain open, rather than collapse, with the pressures of breathing.

Your baby is 21 cm (8.4 in) long and weighs 630 gm (22 oz.). It is amazing to think that something the size of an ear of corn could possibly survive!

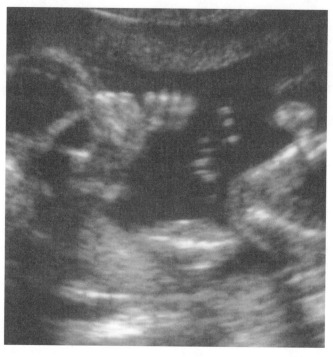

"Thumb sucking is comforting, even while baby is still inside you. Babies have been seen sucking their thumbs from early in the second trimester."

What You Are Doing

Your uterus continues to grow, and is about 4 cm (the width of about three fingers) above your increasingly shallow belly button. Changes are continuing that you can't see, too. Your cholesterol and triglyceride levels increase, albumin (a form of protein) levels decrease (which may contribute to swelling), and your metabolic rate is peaking. You probably still feel pretty good, although round ligament stretching may be increasing.

Special Considerations

No one wants to deliver a premature baby, but those of us who are over 35 are at increased risk for this complication. While the overall incidence of preterm birth is low (6.1 percent), it is 4 times as high as in women aged 20–25. Low-birthweight babies (< 2500 gm or 5 lbs. 7 oz.) are born to roughly 8 percent of over-35-year-olds, compared to 3.6 percent of younger women.

There are several reasons why our older age increases the odds of an early delivery: we have complications like high blood pressure and diabetes more often, both of which may necessitate early delivery. High blood pressure, in particular, may lead to poor growth of the baby and low birthweight. (We'll talk about preterm labor and low birthweight in more detail in week 30.)

What can you expect if your baby is born early? Premature babies, certainly ones born this early, require intensive care to survive. We often talk about survival rates and *morbidity*, or long-term complication rates, when discussing babies who are born too soon. Some babies will survive, only to have significant problems because of their prematurity. Table 24.1 lists the survival and morbidity rates for various ages. We have learned so much and have such wonderful technology today that more and more babies survive with fewer complications. Good follow-up and therapy throughout infancy and childhood may also minimize the impact of any complications that do occur.

A premature baby's biggest problem, more pronounced the earlier the baby is born, is immature lungs and respiratory distress syndrome. Because surfactant production is low until a few weeks before delivery, the lungs may collapse from the pressures associated with breathing air. Since the mid-1980s, we have been able to give premature babies artificial surfactant as soon as they are born; this has been one of the most significant advancements in the care of the premature infant. Even with the ability to give surfactant, these babies are not home free—their tiny little muscles are not strong enough to do the work of breathing, so they need to be on ventilators. Unfortunately, even though mechanical ventilation is necessary to save the baby's life, it can damage the lungs, both from the pressures generated by the ventilator as well as the high levels of oxygen required to maintain an adequate concentration of oxygen in baby's circulation. This scarring of the lungs, called *bronchopulmonary dysplasia* (BPD), can lead to long-term oxygen requirements and asthma-like symptoms.

In addition to the respiratory difficulties, a premature baby's immune and gastrointestinal systems are not mature either. Infections pose a threat to this delicate little being. The baby cannot swallow on his own yet, so he must be fed via a tube placed into the stomach or through an IV. Usually by 34 weeks gestation, a baby has enough strength to nurse or suck from a bottle. Premature babies may develop *necrotizing enterocolitis* (NEC), an inflamma-

TABLE 24.1

Survival and Long-Term Disability Rates for Premature Babies

Gestational Age	Survival (%)	Disability (%)
23 weeks	10–35	> 50
24 weeks	40–70	> 50
25 weeks	50–80	16–25
26 weeks	80–90	9–16
27–29 weeks	> 90	< 10
30–33 weeks	> 95	< 5
> 34 weeks	> 98	< 5

tion of the bowel wall that may lead to bowel perforation; babies fed breast milk are less likely to develop NEC than those fed formula. If NEC is suspected, the baby will be given nothing by mouth and antibiotics will be started, but if a bowel perforation is diagnosed, surgery is necessary.

Premature babies are at higher risk for eye damage, too, and are more likely to need glasses at an early age than full-term babies. *Retinopathy of prematurity* (ROP) is a condition in which there is abnormal growth of blood vessels within the eye. Mild cases require no treatment, but severe cases may require laser therapy to prevent outright blindness. ROP is most common in babies born more than 12 weeks early (< 26–28 weeks). Table 24.2 lists some of the complications associated with prematurity.

If your baby is born prematurely, he will most likely spend several days to weeks in a *neonatal intensive care unit* (NICU) under the care of a *neonatologist*. A neonatologist is a pediatrician with special training and expertise in the care of premature and sick babies. Babies in NICUs are often connected to a myriad of machines and monitors; it is amazing that so many devices can be hooked up to such tiny beings. A heart monitor displays the baby's heart rate, EKG, and breathing rate. Blood pressure cuffs are placed to intermittently monitor the baby's blood pressure. A pulse oximeter measures the amount of oxygen in the baby's blood. A temperature probe ensures the baby is neither too cold nor too warm and that the heated bed in which the baby lives is just right. IV lines supply fluids and possibly nutrients, and serve as a means of delivering antibiotics or blood if needed. Some very premature or sick babies will have intravenous lines placed in the blood vessels of the umbilical cord, both to deliver fluids and medications and also to be used to take blood for the many tests such sick babies require. Some babies who are bigger and stronger may have oxygen delivered via tiny tubes that fit in the nostrils, while others will be *intubated* (have a breathing tube placed) and on a ventilator.

TABLE 24.2

Complications Associated with Prematurity

COMMON, ALMOST UNIVERSAL

Apnea

Periods in which the baby stops breathing. Monitors are used to alert you to this. Stimulating the baby usually starts respiration. Often associated with a slowing of the heart rate (bradycardia). Infants grow out of this spontaneously after several months.

Feeding Problems

Immature, weak muscles and lack of coordination make it difficult for a preemie to nurse or sometimes to even feed from a bottle. Usually, babies born after 34 weeks do not have this problem, and those born earlier develop the appropriate skills by the time they reach what would have been 34 weeks had they not been born sooner. Until then, IV nutrition or tube feedings are done.

Jaundice

Increased *bilirubin* in the baby's blood. Caused by increased breakdown of fragile, immature red blood cells and the immature liver's inability to rid the body of these breakdown products efficiently. Treated by placing the baby under special lights to speed reabsorbing of bilirubin. Very high levels of jaundice can lead to brain damage, and an *exchange transfusion* may be necessary.

VERY COMMON

Hernia

Hernias are protrusions of the bowel through an area of weakness in the abdominal cavity. The groin (*inguinal hernia*) and belly button (*umbilical hernia*) are the most common sites in babies.

TABLE 24.2

Hernias are more common in preemies because these openings did not have a chance to close as they normally do before birth. Umbilical hernias usually resolve without any treatment at all in the first year or two of life, but inguinal hernias generally require surgical correction.

Infection

Both because of an immature immune system and the invasive nature of intensive care, with intravenous lines and multiple procedures, the risk of infection is fairly high in a premature baby. Also, a preemie has had less time to get protective antibodies from Mom.

Patent Ductus Arteriosis (PDA)

Pre-birth, blood from the heart enters the pulmonary artery and is then shunted to the aorta via the *ductus arteriosis,* bypassing the lungs (since the baby is not breathing, there is no oxygen in the lungs and no reason for the blood to go there). After birth, the ductus arteriosis closes within the first few hours or days of life. If the ductus arteriosis does not close properly, high pressure from the aorta forces blood into the lungs and makes it harder for the baby to breathe and also makes the heart work harder. Indomethacin is a drug used to medically constrict the PDA; if unsuccessful, surgery is done to tie off this now abnormal connection.

Reflux

Reflux is when stomach contents come back into the esophagus— basically, it is spitting up. This may irritate the esophagus, and because the milk is not being digested, the baby may not grow properly. While it may occur in any infant, it is more common in premature babies because the muscles at the junction of esopha-

TABLE 24.2

gus and stomach are weaker. Smaller, more frequent feeding and positioning the baby on his stomach, with the head of the bassinet elevated, can diminish reflux. *Never* place an infant under the age of 6 months on his stomach without the express orders of your doctor! Sleeping on the stomach may increase the risk of SIDS (crib death).

Respiratory Distress Syndrome (RDS)
Difficult breathing due to immature lungs. Discussed above. Long-term consequences include increased colds and bronchitis in the first 2 years, increased chance of developing asthma and BPD.

Retinopathy of Prematurity (ROP)
As discussed in preceding text, this abnormal growth of blood vessels in the eye is more common in the very premature baby.

Sugar Imbalance
Preemies often have problems maintaining a normal blood sugar. Usually it is low, and feeding corrects it. This is more pronounced if you were diabetic during the pregnancy. In most cases resolves within the first few days to week of life.

LESS COMMOM, BUT MORE SEVERE

Bronchopulmonary Dysplasia (BPD)
This is a long-term lung disease, a scarring caused by severe RDS or pneumonia. Babies with BPD may have difficulty growing. Oxygen supplementation may be required after the baby goes home. Sometimes steroids or inhalers are used as well.

Intraventricular Hemorrhage (IVH)
Bleeding into the fluid-filled ventricles of the brain or the areas near them. There are four grades of IVH: Grade I is confined to a

TABLE 24.2

tiny area; Grade II extends into the ventricles; in Grade III there is enough blood in the ventricles that they are larger than usual; and in Grade IV, there is blood within the brain tissue itself, resulting in brain damage. The earlier the baby is born, the higher the risk of IVH. Grades III and IV may be associated with hydrocephalus, or "water on the brain," which may in turn lead to both physical and mental delays. Grades I and II IVH, the most common, rarely cause any long-term damage.

Necrotizing Lining or Enterocolitis (NEC)
This inflammation leading to destruction of the entire bowel wall is discussed in text preceding.

Periventricular Leukomalacia (PVL)
This softening of the brain tissue results from oxygen deprivation due to poor blood flow. It may be associated with Grades III or IV IVH. PVL is diagnosed by a head ultrasound 4–8 weeks after birth. Both abnormal physical development ("cerebral palsy") and mental retardation occur. More subtle defects such as learning disabilities, poor hand-eye coordination, or behavioral problems may be the only sign of milder cases.

It can be overwhelming to see your baby lying in an incubator with tubes and wires everywhere. Many NICUs have social workers on staff as well as support groups to help you cope with the emotional aspects of having a preemie.

Frequently Asked Questions

Q I am 23 weeks pregnant and my membranes have ruptured. My doctor and the doctor from the intensive care nursery have both talked to me about whether we want them to even try to save the baby. Why are they asking us that?

A *At 23 weeks, your baby is on the cusp of viability. A few 23-weekers may survive, but the chance of long-term disability is high. It is not until the twenty-fourth week that the chance of the baby surviving is above 50 percent. When a baby is this premature, with poor odds of living, the parents are given the option of trying everything versus not intervening at all and being allowed to hold their tiny baby and let Nature take her course. Saving a premature baby is extremely invasive, and when the odds of successful intervention are so low, some parents would rather not subject their babies to such painful, intrusive measures; others want to do everything possible if there is even the remotest chance the baby will make it. In order for you to make the most informed decision, both the obstetrician and the neonatologist must talk frankly to you.*

Q My baby was born prematurely at 27 weeks, and, thankfully, is doing quite well, off the ventilator after almost a month. The nurses in the NICU keep talking about "adjusted age." What is this?

A *Adjusted age is the age your baby would be if she was born at term. Your daughter was born at 27 weeks, is now a month old, so her adjusted age is 31 weeks. This adjusted age is used to gauge how well a preemie is doing. For example, most babies born after 34 weeks will not need to be on a ventilator because they are strong enough to breathe on their own (they still may need oxygen, though), so a baby born earlier than that would be expected to be off the ventilator by 34 weeks, adjusted age.*

The adjusted age is used for the first year or two of life. Most 3-month-old babies can lift their heads up when they are placed on their stomachs, but when your baby is 3 months old, it will be a week before her original due date, and you would not expect a brand new baby to do that! We use the adjusted age in determining when a preemie should reach certain milestones like holding up the head, rolling over, walking, and talking. By their second birthday, the majority of preemies have caught up, and adjusted age is no longer used.

Week 25

SUN _____ DATE _____

MON _____ DATE _____

TUE _____ DATE _____

WED _____ DATE _____

THUR _____ DATE _____

FRI _____ DATE _____

SAT _____ DATE _____

What Happened This Week?

_____

_____

_____

_____

How I Feel Physically and Emotionally

_____

_____

_____

_____

Bleeding

THERE IS NO sight more terrifying to a pregnant woman than that of blood on her underwear. Once again, we over-35-year-olds are at increased risk for complications such as placenta previa and placental abruption that may lead to bleeding in the second half of pregnancy.

What Baby Is Doing

If exposed to sudden loud noises, your baby may startle—her arms will be thrown wide and then she will curl into a ball in a protective reflex; you may have seen a newborn do the same thing. Your baby's movements are stronger, and if you are relatively thin and if the placenta is on the back wall of your uterus, other people may be able to feel baby move!

Your 25-week baby is 22 cm (8.8 in) long and weighs 725 gm (25.3 oz., or just over 1½ pounds). This is roughly the size of a wedge of watermelon.

What You Are Doing

Your uterus is now the size of a pumpkin. As it grows, it displaces your intestines, leaving less room in your stomach. That, coupled

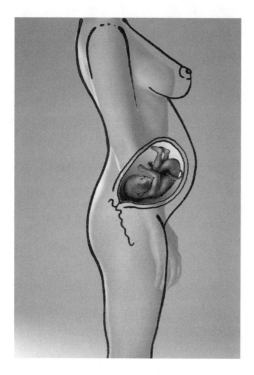

with our old friend progesterone's affect of slowing the emptying of the stomach, may lead to heartburn. Just as it helped with morning sickness in the first trimester, eating frequent small meals may help with the heartburn; overstuff your stomach and you will pay the price with belching and burning.

Your baby is spending about 60 percent of her time in REM sleep, and you begin to follow suit. Many pregnant women report bizarre dreams, like giving birth to a litter of puppies. The increase in REM sleep, however, means there is less time to spend in the more restorative and reparative stages of sleep. You may actually sleep more

You can't hide your 25-week pregnancy! Your breasts are larger and your uterus is above your belly button. You are probably feeling your baby move more consistently now, too.

hours, but feel less rested. Of course, waking up at 2 A.M. with heartburn doesn't do much for a restful night's sleep, either!

Special Considerations

Bleeding in the first trimester is bad enough, but bleeding in the second or third trimester is truly terrifying for most women. One cause of bleeding in the latter half of pregnancy is a *placental abruption* (a.k.a. *abruptio placentae* or just plain *abruption*). This is a separation of the placenta from the wall of the uterus, and may be partial or complete. Because your baby relies on the placenta to supply all of her oxygen, a complete placental abruption will kill the baby unless delivery is immediate. A partial abruption may cause enough harm to necessitate early delivery, or, if small, may not adversely affect your baby at all. Most of the time, vaginal bleeding and uterine or back pain will herald an abruption. On evaluation of the baby's heartbeat, evidence of fetal distress is found in 60 percent of cases. While large abruptions may be seen on ultrasound, smaller ones cannot.

> ✎ DOCTOR'S NOTES
>
> The first time my husband felt our daughter move, I think he was a little freaked out by it. Soon, however, he was playing games with her, tapping on my bulging belly and laughing when she would kick his hand. It became a nightly ritual for him to stroke my belly and tell her goodnight and for her to kick that same spot.

Abruption occurs to one degree or another in 1:150–1:200 deliveries. The incidence of placental abruption does increase with age (from 0.4 percent at age 20, to 0.8 percent at 35, to 2 percent after age 40), but the most common precipitating factor is high blood pressure. Premature rupture of the membranes may also lead to an abruption; the mechanism is believed to be that the sudden decrease in volume of the uterus due to the escape of fluid causes the uterus to shrink—the placenta buckles and an area tears away from the uterine wall. Other risk factors are listed in table 25.1. If you have had a placental abruption in a prior pregnancy, the risk of recurrence is increased tenfold.

TABLE 25.1
Risk Factors for Placental Abruption
African-American heritage
Age
Cigarette smoking
Cocaine use
High blood pressure, either chronic or pregnancy-induced
Trauma
Uterine fibroid located behind placenta

If the abruption is small, close monitoring of both you and your baby is instituted. Weekly or twice weekly *non-stress tests* (NST) or *biophysical profiles* are done (these tests are discussed in detail in week 35) to look for signs the baby is not tolerating this small, chronic abruption. Because the entire area of the placenta is not available for transport of oxygen and nutrients, the baby's growth may be impaired; ultrasounds are done periodically to make sure the baby is growing properly. If at any time the baby is compromised, is not growing, or there is evidence the abruption is enlarging, early delivery is accomplished.

Another possible cause of bleeding at this stage of pregnancy or beyond is a placenta previa. This is when the placenta partially or totally covers the cervical opening. During labor, as the cervix thins and dilates, there is inevitable bleeding as the placenta tears away; because of this, a cesarean section is necessary when a placenta previa exists at term. Placenta previa is diagnosed by ultrasound. Very early in pregnancy, when the uterus is small, a placenta previa is not uncommon—there is only so much room, and an edge of the placenta may partially cover the cervix. Most of the time, as the uterus enlarges, the placenta is drawn away from the cervix and follow-up ultrasounds show that the placenta is well away from the cervix; in one study, placenta previa was diagnosed in 25 percent of ultrasounds done at 18 weeks, but by term, only 0.4 percent persisted. Placenta previa complicates 0.3–0.5 percent of all pregnancies. Like many other things we've discussed in this book, placenta previa becomes more common with increasing age—and with increasing number of pregnancies. In women over the age of 35, the incidence of placenta previa is 1 percent, increasing to 2 percent after age 40. Other risk factors for placenta previa are listed in table 25.2.

Bleeding, especially painless bleeding (i.e., not associated with contractions), is the classic presentation of a placenta previa, and this bleeding may be torrential. In the past, this was how most previas were first diagnosed; today most are discovered during a routine 20-week ultrasound. Because a placenta previa is so common early in pregnancy, as long as you have not experienced any bleeding, no restriction or modifications of your activities are required at this point. If the placenta previa is still present after 24–26 weeks, however, pelvic rest and avoidance of strenuous activity are advised. Pelvic rest is mandatory because intercourse or even a pelvic exam can cause heavy bleeding. If bleeding occurs, there are two main scenarios: bleeding so heavy that immediate delivery via cesarean section is required, regardless of how premature your baby is; or self-limited bleeding without signs of fetal distress, where delivery can be delayed until your baby is mature. If you have a placenta previa and are discharged home after an episode of bleeding, immediate transportation to a nearby hospital is a condition of allowing you to go home—if you live far from a hospital with the capability of performing a cesarean section, you may have to remain hospitalized until the baby is delivered.

Cesarean section is the mode of delivery with a placenta previa. Because the chances of bleeding increases the closer you get to your due date (because the odds of going into labor increase), an amniocentesis is often performed between 36 and 37 weeks to ascertain if the baby's lungs are mature; delivery is scheduled once lung maturity is documented. There is a higher risk of you losing blood during a cesarean section when you have a placenta previa, so blood for transfusion must be immediately available. There is also a higher chance the placenta will be abnormally adherent to the uterus (*placenta accreta, placenta increta, placenta percreta*), which in and of itself increases the risk of hemorrhage. In rare instances, if bleeding cannot be controlled by more conservative measures, an immediate hysterectomy may become necessary. I have delivered more than 2,500 babies in my career, and have had to do two hysterectomies for uncontrollable bleeding at the time of a cesarean section for placenta previa.

TABLE 25.2

Risk Factors for Placenta Previa

Age > 35

Cigarette smoking

Multiple prior pregnancies

Prior cesarean section

Prior uterine surgery like D&C or myomectomy (removal of a
fibroid from the uterine wall)

Twins or more

Frequently Asked Questions

Q A placenta previa was diagnosed on my routine 20-week ultrasound. The doctor repeated the ultrasound today, at 26 weeks, and the placenta previa is still there. Today she told me not to have sex. Why, and why did she just tell me this now?

A *Because the placenta covers the internal opening of the cervix, there is a chance that the impact of a penis on this area could lead to tearing of blood vessels and bleeding. Very early in pregnancy, the cervix is longer, the lower uterine segment is thicker, and sex is less likely to lead to bleeding.*

In addition to avoiding sex, you should not place anything into your vagina—and you should tell any new doctor you have a placenta previa before allowing a pelvic exam. Even an exam can cause blood vessels under the placenta to tear, producing a potentially massive amount of bleeding.

Q I had a placental abruption with my first pregnancy and had to have an emergency cesarean section at 35 weeks. My son is now 5 years old and fine, but I am so afraid of it happening again! What can I do to lessen the chance of a repeat abruption?

A *First, I have to ask why you had an abruption the first time around. If you smoked, for example, not doing so this time is one sure-fire way to lower the risk. Ditto for use of drugs like cocaine. If you had high blood pressure, that could have been the cause; controlling your blood pressure with bed rest, relaxation techniques, or medication can lower the chance of having an abruption.*

Your doctor will probably monitor you more closely this time around. You may have non-stress tests performed weekly, starting after the twenty-eighth week, in order to see if there is any sign of a small separation. Unfortunately, because an abruption can occur rapidly and without warning, monitoring often is not able to predict an impending abruption. The best bet is to eliminate as many risk factors (listed in table 25.1) as possible.

Week 26

SUN _____ DATE _____

MON _____ DATE _____

TUE _____ DATE _____

WED _____ DATE _____

THUR _____ DATE _____

FRI _____ DATE _____

SAT _____ DATE _____

What Happened This Week?

_____

_____

_____

_____

How I Feel Physically and Emotionally

_____

_____

_____

_____

Working Nine to Five

WHEN OUR MOTHERS had us, most of them probably stayed at home throughout most, if not all, of their pregnancies. Today, the vast majority of us work outside the home while we are pregnant, and we want to make sure our work environments do not harm our babies, either through chemical exposure, physical demands, or mental stress.

What Baby Is Doing

Although more and more fat is being deposited every day, your baby still appears lean. The skin is red and wrinkled, as if it is a suit of clothing two sizes too big. Fingernails have formed and extend near the fingertips; by the time she is born, your baby may need her first manicure!

Taste buds have developed by now, and even pre-birth babies show a preference for sweets. Ultrasound studies, ingeniously designed, reveal that exposure to bitter tastes will cause the baby to grimace! I'm not sure whether she liked it or not, but a spicy Thai or Mexican meal would make my daughter much more active.

From My Journal

"9/5/98. Went to Sac [Sacramento] 2 days ago for a growth scan—you were kicking and it was such a trip to feel you move and see it on the screen at the same time. I can't describe the feeling. You weighed 847 gm. . . . "

This is the last week of the second trimester—hard as it may be to believe, your pregnancy is two-thirds over! Your baby is 23 cm (9.2 in) long, from crown to rump. She weighs 820 gm (28.7 oz. = 1 lb. 12 oz.). As the baby gets bigger, I'm having a hard time maintaining the food analogy theme, but this is about as big as a loaf of home-made zucchini bread (currently the only way my daughter will even eat zucchini!).

What You Are Doing

At this point, you have probably gained around 15 pounds, give or take a couple of pounds. The baby accounts for only 2 pounds of this, the uterus and amniotic fluid for another 2 or so pounds, the placenta for a half-pound, your breasts for a bit more than half a pound (although I bet they feel a lot bigger than that!), and an additional few ounces here and there. The majority of the weight is from the fat your body is storing in preparation for nursing a baby later. Your uterus continues to grow at the rate of a centimeter a week.

You may start to notice occasional, irregular, mild tightenings of your uterus, the so-called *Braxton Hicks contractions*. These should be relatively pain free. Named after the man who first described this phenomenon in 1872 (J. Braxton Hicks), these do not cause the cervix to dilate. In the last few weeks of pregnancy, the intensity and frequency of Braxton Hicks contractions do pick up and they may account for false labor.

Special Considerations

Some of us want to work, and some of us have to work. Some of us have jobs we'd leave in a heartbeat given the chance, and some of us have careers we have worked long and hard to build. We are teachers and bankers and maids and lawyers and clerks and bus drivers and secretaries and, yes, even ob-gyns! Most women will be able to continue to work throughout pregnancy, but others may have to stop because of either pregnancy-related complications or the specific nature of their jobs. Many women will need to make some adjustments in their work routine in order to accommodate the physical, emotional, and mental changes that accompany pregnancy.

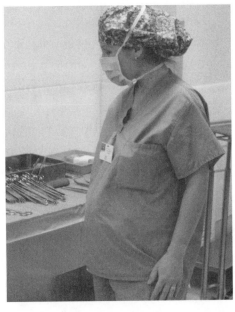

"An operating nurse, Sandy, makes sure all the instruments are in order."

You cannot be forced out of your job merely because you are pregnant. The Pregnancy Discrimination Act of 1978 requires that your pregnancy be treated like any other medical disability. If your employer provides disability coverage for a broken leg, for example, then similar coverage must be extended to you for pregnancy. If your employer makes accommodations for an employee who needs "light duty" due to a back injury, for instance, then you must be allowed light duty as well if your doctor deems it necessary. On the other hand, if your employer does not provide any type of disability for any conditions, pregnancy-related disability is not required, either. Basically, the Pregnancy Discrimination Act demands that you are treated no differently than any other employee.

Some accommodations may need to be made because you are pregnant. If your job requires heavy lifting, your doctor may give you a note restricting lifting to no more than 25–30 pounds in early pregnancy and no more than 15–20 pounds in the third trimester. If you stand in one place for long periods of time, you should be allowed to either sit on a stool for part of your shift or take a 10–15 minute break every couple of hours (put your feet up during these breaks). Women whose jobs require a lot of standing should definitely invest in good maternity support hose. A few jobs, in which exposure to hazardous materials is unavoidable, are completely incompatible with pregnancy, and your doctor may place you on disability as soon as you become pregnant.

A lot of women want to stop working as soon as they learn they are pregnant. Certainly, it is your right to make that choice, but

THE ART OF JUGGLING

Since most of us don't have the luxury of not working during pregnancy, we have to learn how to juggle our pregnancy needs with our employment requirements.

Tracy, age 39: "I travel a lot, and I'm wiped out after a trip, but so far I haven't had to cut back at all."

Marie, age 38: "I'm lucky—my employer is very flexible, so they don't mind if I come in late; it's getting harder and harder to get to work by 8 AM!"

Dru, age 35: "My co-workers and boss are great. I have an administrative job, so I don't have to worry about the physical demands. It's really not been a problem."

don't expect your doctor to write a note excusing you from work and justifying a medical disability if neither the conditions of your job nor complications of your pregnancy make it imperative that you quit. I will do whatever I can to ensure that your working conditions are safe for the baby and as comfortable for you as possible, but I will not lie and say you are incapable of working just because you are pregnant. Pregnancy in and of itself is not a disability.

If you are planning to work during your pregnancy, you will need to evaluate your company's maternity leave policy. Laws vary from state to state; for information, contact your state's labor department or the human resources office at your company. Some states allow 2 to 4 weeks of disability without a medical excuse prior to delivery and an additional 6 weeks after you give birth, while others do not provide for any non-medically mandated leave before your baby is born. The Family and Medical Leave Act (FMLA), signed into federal law on August 5, 1993, mandates that companies employing more than 50 employees in a 75-mile radius allow up to 12 weeks of unpaid leave for the birth or adoption of a child or to care for a sick family member. Your position, or an equivalent one, is guaranteed to be available when you return, and your health benefits are continued while you are out. This law applies to both mothers and fathers. In order to be eligible, the employee must have worked for the company for at least one year and at least 1,250 hours over the past year. Small businesses are exempt from the law, and if you are in the top 10 percent of earners in the company, your employer does not have to honor the FMLA. The FMLA is *unpaid* leave, so you should explore whether your employer or your state provides disability pay while you are on maternity leave. Usually this is less than your normal wages.

If your pregnancy is uncomplicated, you can continue to work right up to the end—my rule of thumb is that you can keep working until your due date or labor, whichever comes first! If you are entitled to a week or two off prior to baby's arrival, and you want to

TEN TIPS FOR WORKING MOMS-TO-BE

1. Find a place at work where you can lie down. Use this during breaks.

2. When sitting at your desk, elevate your legs on an overturned wastebasket.

3. If you sit most of the day, get up and stretch or walk around for 5 minutes every hour.

4. If you stand most of the day, sit and elevate your legs for 10–15 minutes every two hours.

5. If you stand in one place for most of the day, keep a low box or stool nearby (a fat telephone book works, too) and alternate placing one foot on it.

6. Drink an 8-ounce cup of water every 2–3 hours.

7. Empty your bladder at least every 2 hours.

8. Keep nutritious snacks in your desk drawer and eat something every 1–2 hours. Apples, bananas, oranges, dried fruit and nuts, crackers, pretzels, and peanut butter are a few easy-to-stock snacks.

9. Schedule your doctor's appointments for first thing in the morning or last appointment of the day; stay late or come in early to make up for the time off. Some doctors' offices offer weekend or evening appointments.

10. Wear loose, comfortable maternity clothes. Borrow from a friend who has had a baby recently, or try a consignment shop as a way to save money.

take advantage of that, by all means do so. I worked full-time, taking calls and delivering babies right to the end—I delivered my last baby 5 days before mine was born, did my last surgery 3 days before, and saw patients in the office the afternoon before I went into the hospital to have my daughter. I must admit, if I had it to do over again, I would have taken a couple of days off just to relax before taking on the rigors of first-time motherhood!

Frequently Asked Questions

Q I had to have a cerclage placed because of an incompetent cervix, and I am doing very well. However, my doctor has told me not to work more than 30 hours per week (no more than 8 hours in any one day) and to keep off my feet. My boss is not being very helpful in allowing me to rearrange my duties and hours. I need the income, and I don't know what to do!

A *The health of your baby is the most important thing, and you must do whatever it takes to ensure that. Sometimes that means going out on pregnancy-related disability if your employer cannot or will not make accommodations for you. Before you give up on your boss, however, ask your doctor to write a detailed note to your boss explaining exactly what you can and can't do. Have the doctor include a line to the effect that if accommodations cannot be made, she will place you on disability and your boss will have to train someone else to take your place. If your boss realizes he may lose you, he may be more willing to make a few adjustments to keep you—and your expertise— on at least a part-time basis.*

Q After a full day on the job (I'm a postal clerk), I notice my uterus tightens up. This lasts for a couple of hours and it isn't painful. What is this?

A *It sounds like you are having Braxton Hicks contractions. Many women will notice them at the end of the day. As long as they* are mild and irregular, and they go away if you rest and drink extra fluids, they are of no concern. If you can get off your feet a few times a day (ask if you can sit at a tall stool when you are working the post office counter) and drink the recommended eight 8-ounce glasses of water a day, you may not have as many Braxton Hicks contractions in the evening. Contractions that are painful or regular (at this point, even something every 15–20 minutes should be reported to your doctor) must be evaluated.

Q I am a musician and I'm worried about whether the noise could hurt my baby.

A Wow, you're a singer in a rock and roll band! I always wanted to do that but, well, let's just say only my toddler thinks I have a good voice! Exposure to noise louder than 90 decibels has been associated with lower birthweight. This does not mean you have to put away the microphone, however. Turning the volume down is one option. Rearranging the speakers and your relationship to them is another. Limiting your time on-stage is a third way to reduce the amount of noise your baby is exposed to. When you are not performing, take it easy, and make sure your diet is stellar.

Be sure your doctor knows what you do for a living. She may want to get periodic ultrasounds to make sure your baby is growing appropriately. If there is any sign of poor growth, or if you notice a marked decrease in your baby's normal activity patterns after you perform, you may have to put your performances on hold for the sake of your baby.

Q Why are so many pregnancy complications higher when we are older? It doesn't seem fair!

A I know it can be frightening to read all these statistics about how age is a risk factor for one bad thing and another. Age is a risk, for the most part, because other underlying conditions for a given *complication increase in the general population as a function of increasing age. For example, in the case of placental abruption, it is not so much that you reach 35 and all of a sudden your placenta is going to leap off the uterine wall as it is that high blood pressure, the primary cause of abruption, is more likely to be found in a 40-year-old than a 25-year-old. In the majority of cases, what I said earlier in this book holds true—a healthy older mom-to-be is going to have less complications than an obese, pack-a-day smoking, junk-food eating twenty-something. And I'd rather take care of that conscientious, motivated-42 year-old!*

Week 27

SUN _____ DATE

MON _____ DATE

TUE _____ DATE

WED _____ DATE

THUR _____ DATE

FRI _____ DATE

SAT _____ DATE

What Happened This Week?

_____

_____

_____

How I Feel Physically and Emotionally

_____

_____

_____

It's a Boy and a Girl and . . .

B ECAUSE WE ARE older moms, more of us will have had to use high-tech means to conceive—and this increases the odds we will bring more than one baby home from the hospital. Even those of you who were not "fertility challenged" are more likely to conceive twins (or more!) merely as a function of age. It doesn't seem quite right—we are older and Mother Nature expects us to nurse two (or more) babies, and change two (or more) sets of diapers and run after two (or more) toddlers at once!

What Baby Is Doing

Your baby, once a tiny ball of cells, has now entered the third and final trimester of her life inside you. All of her major organ systems are fully functional, although they still have significant maturation to go. Brain growth explodes in these last three months.

At 24 cm (9.6 in) long and 910 gm (31.8 ounces, just shy of 2 pounds) your baby is the size of that loaf of zucchini bread from last week, plus a slice of banana bread! I think I'm going to have to forgo the food analogies from this point on, because baby is getting too big to be compared to the contents of my refrigerator!

What You Are Doing

You have probably enjoyed the last several weeks of your pregnancy, the so-called honeymoon period of the second trimester. The third trimester you are now entering is a time of physical and emotional upheaval for many women. As your belly gets bigger and bigger, discomforts like lower backache may increase. You may feel both anxious to have the baby out and fearful of just what exactly you are supposed to do with this little person who is completely dependent on you to meet all his needs.

You may notice you are becoming more short of breath, especially at night. As your uterus expands and displaces your intestines upward, you may feel as if you just can't take in a good breath; this is much more exaggerated when lying down. You may need to find creative sleeping arrangements; many moms-to-be spend the night in the La-Z-Boy recliner.

Special Considerations

Thanks to the same technology that has allowed some of us even to have babies, more of us are having twins, triplets, or even higher. Comparing the years 1980–1982 with 1995–1997, the rate of twin births jumped 63 percent for women aged 40–44 and 1,000 percent for women 45–49; more twins were born to women aged 45–49 in 1997 alone than were born in the entire decade of the 1980s! In 1997, the number of multiple births in the United States was 110,874; the overwhelming majority were twins (104,137), but more and more triplets (6,148), quadruplets (510), and quintuplets and greater (79) were born. Women 35 and older accounted for almost 20 percent of the twins, and an amazing 68 percent of the triplets and above! This high number of multiple births can be attributed to the use of fertility drugs and assisted reproductive technologies like IVF.

The overall incidence of *identical (monozygotic) twins* world-

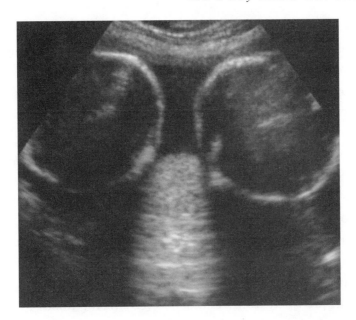

"Two heads are better than one. Here, twins put their heads together—probably plotting mischief for after they are born."

wide is 4:1,000, and is independent of age, race, number of prior pregnancies (*parity*), and heredity. Identical twins occur when one egg is fertilized and then splits into two separate babies. The incidence of *fraternal* (*dizygotic*) *twins* varies considerably by country, ranging from 1:1,000 in Japan to 7:1,000 in white Americans to 11:1,000 in African-Americans to a whopping 49:1,000 in Nigeria! Fraternal twins come from two different eggs fertilized by two different sperm and are no more alike than any other siblings. The rate of fraternal twins is remarkably influenced by age, race, parity, heredity, and, obviously, use of fertility drugs. The rates of multiple births quoted reflect the numbers at delivery; with the advent of earlier and earlier ultrasounds, we now know many more twins are conceived, only to have one lost early on. Miscarriage of one of a set of twins (or more) may account for some cases of first-trimester vaginal bleeding in which subsequent ultrasound shows one healthy baby.

Why—and how much—does the incidence of fraternal twins

increase with age? Well, for one thing, as we get older ovulation becomes more irregular; some months you may not ovulate at all and others you will release more than one egg. One reason for releasing more eggs as we get older is that time is running out for us to reproduce, so Mother Nature wants more than one egg out there for sperm to find in order to increase the odds you will get pregnant and continue the species. As for how much more likely you are to have twins (or more), based on 1997 U.S. data, 2 percent of 20–24-year-olds delivered twins or more; by age 35–39, that more than doubles, to 4.3 percent, and among 45–54-year-old women, 16.6 percent delivered two or more babies! Of course, part of that huge number in the oldest group of women is attributable to a higher percentage of them undergoing fertility treatments. The odds of a multiple birth from *clomiphene* (*Clomid*) is about 5 percent, virtually all of them twins. With injected *gonadotropins* (*Pergonal, Fertinex, Follistim*), the multiple pregnancy rate ranges from 10 to 30 percent, with as many as 5 percent triplets or more. By an unknown mechanism, gonadotropins also increase the odds of identical twins by as much as threefold.

Carrying more than one baby provides a special set of challenges—for you and for your babies (and for the entire family once the babies are born). If you are carrying twins, you will be expected to gain between 40 and 50 pounds. Your blood volume will increase more than with a single baby, and you are more likely to become anemic. Gestational diabetes (discussed in week 28) and high blood pressure (week 34) are more common, too. Because of the load you are carrying, backaches, heartburn, varicose veins, and hemorrhoids are more likely to bother you. It is almost a given that you will not be able to work or engage in all your usual activities for your entire pregnancy.

Miscarriages, especially in identical twins that share the same amniotic sac (*monochorionic twins*) are more common than with singletons. Major birth defects occur in about 2 percent of twins, compared with 1 percent of single babies, and minor defects are also more common (4 percent compared to 2.5 percent). Twins or higher are much, much more likely to be smaller than their single-ton counterparts, even if born at the same gestational age. The average birthweight at term for a singleton is 3,600 gm (7 lbs. 13 oz.), but for a twin it is 3,000 gm (6½ lbs.). Preterm birth is more likely as well. The average gestational age at delivery is 36 weeks in twins, 32 weeks in triplets, and 30 weeks in quadruplets.

If you are carrying more than one baby, your pregnancy is considered high risk, and you will be monitored closely. You need 300 calories per baby above your pre-pregnancy requirements. You need extra iron (60–100 mg/day) and folate (1 mg/day) as well. Beginning at 20 weeks, you will have an ultrasound monthly to make sure all babies are growing adequately. If there is any discordance between the babies, monitoring will be instituted (see week 35). If you have triplets or more, your progress will probably be followed by a perinatologist in addition to your regular obstetrician. Bed rest will probably be a fact of life if you are carrying more than twins.

Not only does carrying multiple babies pose special challenges throughout pregnancy, it does so in the delivery room too. Virtually all triplets and higher are delivered by cesarean section. Twins may be delivered vaginally if the first twin is head down, but if he is breech, then a cesarean section is planned. Sometimes the first baby delivers without difficulty, but the second one, by virtue of position, fetal distress, or bleeding, requires a cesarean section. If you are carrying more than one baby, forget those visions of delivering in the homey, dimly lit birthing room; you will have your babies in an operative delivery room, with (usually) two obstetricians and one person skilled in caring for infants (pediatrician, family practitioner, neonatal nurse) present for each baby, plus an anesthesiologist (in case an emergency cesarean is required), and a nurse or two to help the delivering doctor(s). It may sound like a three-ring circus, but it is still the miracle of birth, and you won't care that you couldn't have soft lights and music when you hold your babies in your arms.

Frequently Asked Questions

Q My mother was a twin and I am a twin, too. My husband has a twin sister. I am 42 and this is my fourth pregnancy. And, I conceived on Clomid! I guess we are going to have twins, huh?

A *Well, you might lose a few dollars if you bet on it, but you certainly have a good chance of having twins. Based on your age and the number of children you have already had, the chance you conceived twins is 7–8 percent. Clomid leads to twins in roughly 5 percent of cases. You being a twin means the odds you are having twins is 1.7 percent; your husband being a twin only increases the chance by 0.8 percent. All told, your chance of having twins is about 15 percent. Remember, this is compared to an average rate of <3 percent!*

Q Everyone is so excited we are having triplets. That is, everyone but me. What is wrong with me?

A *There is nothing wrong with you. I'd be petrified, too. Very few of us wish for triplets; our dreams tend to run to one perfect, chubby-cheeked, laughing baby who sleeps through the night from birth, who we push through the park to the admiring* oohs *and* aahs *from all around. First, there are the increased complications associated with carrying three babies, not only in terms of the high chance of preterm birth, but also the physical discomfort you are probably experiencing. Next, there is the concern about exactly how you are going to take care of three babies at once. The answer to the second concern is to ask for help—frequently and loudly, and starting now. You cannot do it by yourself, and even if your husband pitches in 100 percent, you will still need outside help at least for cleaning, running errands, and so on. Once you deliver and the babies are home and healthy, I can guarantee you one thing: When you push them through the park in their triple stroller, you will be the center of attention, and you will be beaming as you show off your darling triplets.*

Q I'm having twins, and we are so excited. I nursed my other two children, and I plan to nurse these babies as well. Any hints for successful breastfeeding of twins?

A *The cardinal rule for successful nursing is to take care of yourself. In order to meet the demands of two babies, you will need to eat a super-healthy diet and drink lots of fluids—and get as much rest as you can (this means letting someone else do the household chores, or learning to love dust bunnies). Some nursing moms prefer to nurse the babies separately, but most find it more efficient to feed both together. If you do nurse them separately, alternate which baby gets to go first, so both get their fair share of both foremilk and hindmilk (see week 36 for a full discussion of breastfeeding). You can hold them so their bodies lie across one another, or use the football hold, with heads resting on a pillow and bodies stretched along your sides, feet near your back. Using a pillow to help support the babies not only helps avoid back, neck, and arm strain, but also frees up your hands so you can eat a snack, drink some water, or even read a child care book! The laws of supply and demand generally work so that you will produce enough milk to keep both babies happy, healthy, and growing on schedule. If you cannot supply enough milk to satisfy two hungry babies or if you choose to supplement with formula to (1) give yourself a break, or (2) allow Daddy special bonding time with the babies, then alternate nursing one while someone else gives the other a bottle. Breastfeeding twins can be challenging, but mothers I know who have done it find it incredibly rewarding.*

Week 28

SUN _____ DATE

MON _____ DATE

TUE _____ DATE

WED _____ DATE

THUR _____ DATE

FRI _____ DATE

SAT _____ DATE

What Happened This Week?

_____

_____

_____

_____

How I Feel Physically and Emotionally

_____

_____

_____

_____

Too Sweet

Diabetes, either pre-existing or developed during pregnancy, is another of those things we over-35-year-olds have to contend with more often than do our younger counterparts. Due to advances in diagnosis and treatment, diabetes in pregnancy is not the catastrophic development it was in the early 1900s, when most diabetic women could not conceive, and those few who did had only a 40 percent chance of their babies surviving. As recently as the 1970s, women with pre-existing diabetes were advised not to become pregnant; if they did, they were told the risks were so great they should consider terminating the pregnancy. Times have changed, and we and our children are the beneficiaries.

What Baby Is Doing

After weeks of being closed, your baby's eyes open this week. Thin, short eyelashes frame the eyes, which are usually blue; final eye color does not develop until several months after birth. If you are carrying a boy, his testicles will begin to descend into his scrotum this week.

233

Your baby is aware of much that goes on outside of his watery home. Research has shown that babies can learn the rudiments of language while still in utero; a baby's cry in its very rhythm often matches the cadence and intonations of his mother's voice. Babies can learn to recognize certain songs and poems as well. In a study done in France in the mid-1990s, mothers recited a nursery rhyme 3 times a day from 33 to 37 weeks, and the babies heartbeats were monitored. By the time the study ended, the babies' heart rates differed depending on whether Mom recited the familiar nursery rhyme or a new one during the monitoring sessions! I read *Oh, Baby, the Places You'll Go,* an adaptation of Dr. Seuss, to Hunter every night for the last two months of my pregnancy. After her birth, when I would read this book she would quiet down and look at me, as if to say, "I remember this!"

Your baby is now 25 cm (10 in) from crown to rump and 35 cm (14 in) from head to toe. He weighs 1,000 gm (2 lbs. 3 oz.).

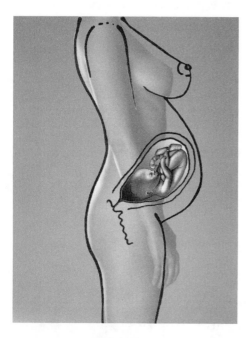

At 28 weeks, you may begin to notice a bit of backache thanks to your burgeoning belly.

What You Are Doing

Up until this point, you have probably been seeing your doctor every month; starting now, visits will increase to every 2 weeks. The twenty-eighth week is the most common time to have a glucose test to rule out *gestational diabetes,* discussed in detail later in this chapter, and to have the RhoGam shot if you are Rh negative. A blood count to check for anemia may be done as well.

Your uterus is well above your belly button, taking up

From My Journal

"9/13/98. 27⁵/₇ weeks. I love how you kick me when I go to bed at night, or when I'm listening to some other baby's heartbeat in the office. I love being pregnant with you, and hope I am providing a good and healthy home for you. I want you to grow big and strong and deliver at term, happy and healthy. I want the best for you throughout your life. You are the center of my world now—and Jeff's too—but we will do our best not to overpower you, to give you the freedom to explore the world on your own. We hope to give you a solid basis for making responsible decisions. We will support you in whatever paths you choose in life. We will—and already do—love and cherish you. We will do our best, but mistakes will be made along the way, as we learn to be parents. We will all learn and laugh and love together."

about three-quarters of the space in your abdomen. While most women experience slow and steady growth of the uterus—a centimeter a week at this stage—others seem to pop out overnight. You may be uncomfortable in your body, but you have probably gotten used to the whole idea of being pregnant and are looking forward to the time when your baby is in your arms.

Special Considerations

Diabetes is the most common medical complication of pregnancy, occurring in approximately 2.5–3 percent of all births; the vast majority (90 percent) of these represent gestational diabetes, or diabetes first diagnosed during pregnancy. Gestational diabetes is detected by a *glucose tolerance test,* commonly referred to as the "glucola" test, done between 24 and 28 weeks. If you have risk factors (table 28.1) other than age alone, you may be screened in the first trimester as well; even if the result early in pregnancy was normal, you need to be re-screened now. The glucola test involves drinking a special beverage (often cola flavored, hence the name!) containing exactly 50 gm of glucose. Blood is drawn exactly 1 hour after the drink is finished; if the blood sugar level is > 140 mg/dl, the screening test is considered positive, and a more definitive test, the 3-hour glucose tolerance test (3-hour GTT) is done. Unlike the screening glucola, for the 3-hour GTT you do need to be fasting: blood is drawn while you are fasting, then you are given a drink containing 100 gm of glucose, then blood is drawn 1, 2, and 3 hours afterward. If you have two abnormal results on the 3-hour GTT, gestational diabetes is diagnosed. Table 28.2 indicates normal values for the 3-hour GTT. Some women feel nauseated from the very sweet drink and may even throw up. If this occurs, an accurate result cannot be obtained, and the test will need to be repeated. One study showed that 18 Jelly Belly jelly beans could be substituted for the drink. Ask your doctor about this alternative.

If gestational diabetes is diagnosed, dietary management is begun in hopes of keeping sugar levels < 105 when fasting and < 120 when measured 2 hours after a meal. Depending on both your blood sugar levels and your doctor's preferences, these levels are monitored either weekly in your doctor's office or daily by you. Monitoring is done by a finger stick; the drop of blood obtained is captured on a test strip and placed into a *glucometer,* a small, easy-to-use device that measures blood sugar. If sugar levels cannot be controlled by diet and moderate exercise alone, *insulin* therapy is begun. Insulin is injected from 1 to 4 times a day, based on sugar levels. If sugar levels are kept within the recommended ranges, either by diet or by insulin, complications to you and your baby are low. If you need insulin, you will have fetal testing done (discussed in depth in week 35). (A study released in the fall of 2000 suggests that oral diabetes medication may be safe and effective in treating gestational diabetes; as I write this, however, use of such medication is far from standard.) After delivery, sugar levels usually return to normal rapidly, but women with gestational diabetes have a 50 percent chance of developing overt diabetes within 20 years. You should periodically be screened, first with a 2-hour GTT 6 weeks after delivery (or after breastfeeding is stopped), and if that is normal, with yearly fasting blood sugars.

Diabetes that exists prior to pregnancy can have a profound impact on both mother and baby. It is vitally important that all women with diabetes who are considering pregnancy have a pre-conception visit with their doctors. Because of the potential for oral diabetes drugs to adversely affect your baby, a transition to insulin ideally is made as soon as you begin attempting pregnancy, and definitely as soon as you find out you are pregnant. If your blood sugar is under good control at the time of conception (and remains well controlled throughout), complications are less likely. Prior to pregnancy, a *glycosolated hemoglobin* (HbA1c) is drawn. If HbA1c is normal (between 5 and 8 percent), the risk of birth defects is the same as in the general population (about 3 percent, as you recall from week 9), but if HbA1c is >9.5 percent, the risk for major birth defects jumps to 10–20 percent.

Other potential consequences of poorly controlled diabetes in pregnancy (whether it is pre-existing or gestational) are stillbirth (in women with overt diabetes, the risk increases fourfold), and *macrosomia*. Macrosomia means the baby is big, and this can lead to problems with delivery. Cesarean section is much more likely if your baby is built like an NFL linebacker. Another consequence of macrosomia is *shoulder dystocia*, where the baby's shoulders are so big that they can get stuck behind the pubic bone during a vaginal delivery. This is an obstetric emergency that requires a cool head and a systematic approach to resolve. Shoulder dystocia may lead to stretching and injury of nerves in the baby's neck and shoulder, and subsequent loss of full function in that arm. For the most part, pregnancy does not alter the course of diabetes for you. The main exception to this rule occurs if you already have eye damage as the result of your diabetes. Once again, if your sugars are well controlled, you are less likely to have progressive eye damage as a result of pregnancy.

If you have overt diabetes, you will be monitored very closely during your pregnancy. Not only will you need to check your sugar frequently throughout the day, your obstetrician will likely have you see an optometrist or ophthalmologist to rule out existing eye disease. You will probably see a perinatologist as well and have a targeted ultrasound around 18–20 weeks to look for some of the major birth defects (especially heart defects) that are more common in diabetics. Ultrasound will be done every 4–6 weeks after 24 weeks to make sure your baby is growing appropriately, neither too big

TABLE 28.1

Risk Factors for Gestational Diabetes

Age > 25 (risk steadily increases with age, rising from 0.8 percent at ages <20 to 6.6 percent of women 40–49)

Diabetes in close family member

Ethnic background: Hispanic/Latina; Native American; Asian; Indian; African-American; Pacific Islander

Gestational diabetes with a prior pregnancy

Obesity

Prior delivery of a baby > 9 pounds

TABLE 28.2	
Screening	Blood Glucose Level (mg/dl)
1 hour	< 140
3-Hour GTT	
Fasting	< 105
1 hour	< 190
2 hour	< 165
3 hour	< 145

nor too small. You will definitely undergo testing for your baby's well-being beginning between 28 and 32 weeks. You are more likely to develop high blood pressure along with your diabetes and may need to be delivered early. If you have not gone into labor on your own by your due date, your labor will be induced, because the risk of harm to your baby increases after the fortieth week. While this all sounds very scary, the majority of women with diabetes—and their babies—do well with good prenatal care.

Frequently Asked Questions

Q I am 39 and pregnant with my third child. My sister is diabetic, and I had gestational diabetes with my son (now 6 years old), so my doctor had me do the glucola test at the first prenatal visit. It was normal then, so why do I have to repeat it now?

A *Pregnancy is a time of change both externally (as you well know from your evolving profile) and internally. In all pregnant women, insulin production by the pancreas is increased, beginning in the first trimester, and production of glucose by the liver is increased in the late second trimester in order to ensure that your baby's needs for sugar are being met. Early in pregnancy, due to increased insulin production, your body may be able to respond normally to a glucose challenge, and you will have a normal result on the glucola. Later in pregnancy, levels of hormones that promote a diabetic state increase, your liver churns out more glucose, and your body becomes more resistant to the effects of insulin, all in an effort to keep a steady supply of glucose to your baby. If you are producing more glucose than average, or not enough insulin, or your body is extra-resistant to the insulin you are making, you will "flunk" the glucola and 3-hour GTT. This is why a normal test early in pregnancy does not mean you will continue to respond normally and why a glucola is done around 28 weeks, shortly after insulin resistance begins.*

From My Journal

"I picture you as a little girl, with straight brown hair [I was wrong, at least so far—Hunter is a real towhead] and clear blue-gray eyes [100 percent on the mark]. You are strong and feisty [that is an understatement as my daughter nears her second birthday]. I had an image of you in hockey gear—street or ice, I'm not sure. You can be and do anything. . . . "

Q I'm not due for another 12 weeks, but I'm having incredibly vivid dreams about the baby—not about giving birth, but about him being here, and me changing diapers and singling lullabies—and he's three feet tall and talks! Is this weird, or what?

A *Many moms-to-be, especially in the third trimester, have Technicolor dreams about what their baby is going to be like. As the time of delivery approaches, we become impatient and want to meet this child, so dreams about what the baby will look like are common. Imagining the baby being born full-grown may relate to fears about having to care for a tiny, helpless newborn—heck, if your baby were born able to talk, you wouldn't have to struggle to figure out if that cry means he's hungry, or wet, or bored, or just in need of a cuddle.*

Q I have been diabetic since I was 11. I had two miscarriages in my twenties, but I was wild and irresponsible and often didn't take my insulin. Now I am 36, in a new marriage, and am petri-fied that something will happen to this baby. I've done everything I can to stay healthy, give myself insulin 3 times a day, check my sugars 5 or 6 times a day, and my HbA1c runs around 7 percent.

A *You are doing everything you should, and your sugar control, as reflected in that normal HbA1c, is excellent. You have probably already had the targeted ultrasound to rule out major birth defects, and maybe even a CVS or amniocentesis due to your age. Your doctor will have you start fetal monitoring in the next week or so to make sure the baby is doing well. (See week 35 for ways to monitor the baby's health inside your womb.) If you continue to take good care of yourself, and the baby's testing is reassuring, then you can feel very confident that you will bring home a wonderful, healthy baby.*

Week 29

SUN   DATE

MON   DATE

TUE   DATE

WED   DATE

THUR   DATE

FRI   DATE

SAT   DATE

What Happened This Week?

How I Feel Physically and Emotionally

Divide and Conquer

You DID NOT make this baby by yourself (okay, if you are a single mom or used donor sperm you did, but otherwise . . .), so you should not have to take care of this baby by yourself. Asking for help is not a sign of weakness—it is a sign of intelligence! And intelligent women plan, so now's the time to think about how you are going to manage the soon-to-be arriving newest member of the family.

What Baby Is Doing

White fat, important as an energy source, begins to increase and will soon account for almost 4 percent of your baby's total weight. Blood cells are being formed in the spleen, and the immune system is becoming functional. Antibodies that cross the placenta from you to your baby help to protect your baby from infections she may be exposed to shortly after birth, when her system is still immature.

Teeth are still hidden in your baby's gums, but enamel has formed. In 1:2,000 babies, one or two teeth will have already erupted at the time of birth. Because they may cause pain with breastfeeding or may come loose and be inadvertently inhaled, these teeth are usually pulled.

Your baby's crown–rump length is 26 cm (10.4 in) and total height is almost 37 cm (14.8 in). She weighs 1150 gm (2½ lbs.). If born at this point, your baby has a better than 90 percent chance of survival.

What You Are Doing

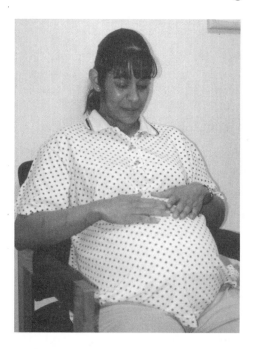

Patricia, age 37, and pregnant with twins, enjoys a quiet moment—she has three children at home already.

If you happen to get your cholesterol checked at this point in your pregnancy, you may be shocked at how high it is. Cholesterol levels increase from an average of 180 pre-pregnancy to near 280 by the time you deliver. Cholesterol is needed in the production of progesterone, which, you have already learned, is sky-high during pregnancy. While you should eat a healthy diet, pregnancy is not the time to try to achieve world record low cholestrol readings! Soon after delivery, however, cholesterol levels return to normal.

Your metabolic rate continues to increase and is at its peak now. You actually require an additional 400 calories daily in order to meet the demands of the third trimester. Your uterus continues to grow at the rate of a centimeter a week, and now measures 29 cm (± 2 cm) above your pubic bone. You should still be gaining about a pound a week.

Special Considerations

Being pregnant can be a tough job, but let me tell you, taking care of a baby is even tougher. You cannot do it on your own. If your significant other is not helping out around the house, now is the time for an equal responsibility rebellion.

While you are still pregnant, you need extra rest. If you are working outside the home, you may return at the end of a long day with swollen ankles—put your feet up and relax and let your partner fix dinner. If you have other children, they are clamoring for your attention when you get home, and you are rushing around trying to pick up toys and get dinner on the table. Order pizza and spend some time reading quietly to your kids. Now is not the time to be Martha Stewart! Even if you are a stay-at-home mom-to-be, if you have kids you need some down time. Make it a habit a few nights a week to have Daddy take the kids for a walk while you soak in the tub—or have the little ones help Daddy make dinner while you go for a solitary walk.

This is the time to start thinking about who is going to do what after the baby is born. If you are working now and this is your first baby, you may think (as I did) that you will have all this free time during your maternity leave to (1) cook gourmet meals, (2) keep the house clean, and (3) write the Great American Novel while your little cherub sleeps. It's a beautiful dream, but it is just that—a dream. You cannot do it all alone, and if you try you will end up an exhausted, depressed new mom. You and your mate should decide now what responsibilities each of you will have, and whether hiring someone to come in and clean the house once a week is a worthwhile investment (Answer: It's one of the best ways to spend $50 I can imagine!). If you are going this pregnancy alone, enlist the help of family and friends. When someone says, "Call me if you need anything," do just that. Ask a few friends to make meals you can freeze, so you don't have to worry about cooking for yourself in those first few weeks after baby is born. Call others up and ask each to make a commitment to watch your baby once every few weeks so you can either take a nice long hot shower or go to the grocery store without baby, baby carrier, and diaper bag in tow. When my best friend had her first child, she called me up one afternoon and asked me to come over just so she could take a shower!

One thing I learned during my pregnancy and the first few months after Hunter was born was that I had to be very specific with my husband. Men (and friends and family) are not mind readers. It is better to give a list of things to do—take out the garbage every Wednesday, go to the grocery store and get the things on this

✎ DOCTOR'S NOTES

It took me a few weeks of trying to be Superwoman and failing miserably before I understood this need to get help. One day, when I was still in my pajamas at 3 P.M., had loads of laundry to do, the baby was crying and so was I, I realized I could not do it all. I remember wailing to my husband, "I went to Bryn Mawr. I'm a doctor! Why can't I do this?" and his reply was, "Because you are human." When I re-hired the cleaning lady, asked my husband to be responsible for food, and I devoted my energies to taking care of Hunter—and me—everything began to run more smoothly and we were all much happier. I never did start writing that novel, but maybe after this book is finished. . . . I hope that reading this before you have your baby will save you some of the anxiety and guilt so many of us needlessly place on ourselves.

list, pick up Junior from daycare at 5:30 and take him to the park for an hour—than to just say you need help. Sit down with your significant other and make a list of all the things that need to be done every week. Take turns choosing one chore (you get to go first because you are pregnant), so that the work is evenly divided. If there is an item that you just cannot do because it is physically too taxing or just too distasteful during pregnancy, put it in your mate's column and choose something else to put in yours (you have to do it this way or no one is going to scrub the toilets, unless you follow my earlier advice and hire someone to clean every week or two). You can even include chores that don't need to be done now but that will become mountainous (like washing clothes) after your baby is born. Children can be included, too. Older children can—and want to be—enormously helpful. Even my toddler can help by picking up her toys or wiping off the table (she loves to "cween de for"—clean the floor). By dividing and conquering, the entire family will benefit, because you will have more time and energy to do fun things together.

Frequently Asked Questions

Q My husband is being wonderful about helping out, but I'm feeling so guilty. I have a wonderful career and am very independent; in fact, I'm the one all my friends turn to for help.

A *The 40 weeks of pregnancy and the first few months after your baby is born are your time to be taken care of. This is the time when you should cash in some of those chips, telling your friends that this time you need their help. This is also the time to learn to stand up for yourself and say "No" when asked to do additional projects at work, plan a neighborhood block party, or serve on the PTA. It is wonderful to give, it is true, but it is also wonderful to be on the receiving end— if you think about it as giving your friends and family the pleasure of doing something for you, it may make being slightly less independent more palatable.*

Q On a recent ultrasound to check the location of the placenta, the technician commented that she saw teeth in the baby's jaw. Is my baby going to be born with a full set of teeth?

A *Seeing the bright echoes of developing teeth on ultrasound does not mean your baby will have a full set of choppers at birth. Both baby teeth and developing permanent teeth are present, buried in the gums, and the enamel covering the teeth may be seen on ultrasound. Natal teeth, those that have erupted at birth, occur only rarely. You will probably not have to deal with your baby teething until 6 months after birth. Even though we saw the tooth buds on a 32-week-ultrasound, my daughter didn't get her first tooth until she was a year old—I was worrying we would have to get miniature dentures made for her!*

Q I am always hot. I sweat, even though it's winter. What can I do about this?

A *Running hot is a consequence of your increased metabolic rate, as is sweating. As your body works hard to nourish your growing baby, excess heat is dissipated through dilated blood vessels in the skin. You perspire more both to rid your body of waste products and, more important, to cool yourself as the perspiration evaporates. Using a good antiperspirant will help keep you dry. Dressing in layers is key—when you get warm, remove a layer or two. Keeping a window open or a fan on to help circulate the air will also help cool you off.*

Q My husband says that since I plan to breastfeed he won't need to get up with the baby at night. I'm feeling like I'm going to have to do everything, and it is making me frustrated and angry.

A *Talk to your husband about your feelings. He may be feeling left out because he can't participate in feeding the baby. Even if you breastfeed, there are a lot of things he can do. If the baby is sleeping in another room, he can get the baby and bring her to you to nurse, or change her diapers. He can hold her and walk with her when she is fussy and nursing is not what she wants or needs. My husband was wonderful at this; even now, if our daughter wakes in the night or won't go to sleep for me, he can get her back to dreamland. This makes him feel great, because it is something he does better than me.*

Week 30

SUN   DATE

MON   DATE

TUE   DATE

WED   DATE

THUR   DATE

FRI   DATE

SAT   DATE

What Happened This Week?

How I Feel Physically and Emotionally

Preterm Labor

PRETERM LABOR, OCCURRING prior to 37 weeks, afflicts roughly 20 percent of pregnancies, resulting in a preterm birth slightly less than 10 percent of the time. Being over 35 increases the odds of a preterm birth, not because of age alone, but because of the other risk factors that are more likely to occur the older we get.

What Baby Is Doing

Your baby's eyes are wide open now and will follow a strong light shining on your belly. If you are sunbathing (wearing a good sunscreen, of course!), your baby sees a warm red-orange glow as the sunlight shines through all the layers of your abdominal wall and uterus. Hair is continuing to grow, and depending on your ethnic background, your baby may have quite the head of hair already. Although baby is filling out, the skin is still somewhat wrinkled.

During this week, baby's bone marrow takes over production of red blood cells from the spleen, although the spleen will continue to be important in white blood cell production. On ultrasound, the chest can be seen to rise and fall off and on. These breathing movements not only help strengthen the muscles used in breathing but are essential for normal lung development; if the baby does not breathe in amniotic fluid, the lungs may be too small to take in an adequate supply of oxygen after birth. Assessment of fetal breathing movements is an important measure of well-being as part of a *biophysical profile* (discussed in detail in week 35).

Tipping the scales at 1,300 gm (2 lbs. 13 oz.), your baby's CRL (crown–rump length) is 27 cm (10.8 in), and she is 37.5 cm (15 in) tall.

What You Are Doing

When your doctor tests your urine in the office, you may have a small amount of sugar or protein in it. Because your urine volume is increased and your kidneys are working faster and harder to filter all the extra fluid circulating throughout your body, a little bit of sugar or protein from your blood can escape into your urine; small amounts of protein (up to 1+ on a visual dipstick) are normal, but larger amounts may be a sign of pre-eclampsia (see week 36). Fluid accumulates outside of the circulatory system as well, peaking at 1.5 extra liters this week. This contributes to the swollen feet and ankles so common in the third trimester.

As your uterus grows, and grows and grows, the two abdominal muscles that run from your lower ribs to your pubic bone may be pulled apart in the middle. This is called *diastasis recti,* and is neither harmful to you or your baby. Your pregnancy is three-quarters over—30 weeks down, 10 to go!

Special Considerations

Preterm labor is contractions occurring prior to 37 weeks that lead to dilation or *effacement* of the cervix. That last part is critical: if the cervix does not dilate or thin out in response to the contractions, then it is not preterm labor but rather *preterm contractions.* Preterm contractions are annoying, and may require an exam every time they occur to make sure that the cervix is not changing, but they do not require treatment. Preterm labor, on the other hand, is treated to diminish the odds of a preterm birth (see week 24 to review the problems associated with prematurity). In 1997, 11.4 percent (423,107) of all births in the United States occurred prior to 37 weeks.

Up until just a few years ago, if your doctor had the slightest suspicion you were starting preterm labor, she would put you on *tocolytics*, medications to stop contractions. Until the cervix begins to change, it is almost impossible to distinguish annoying preterm contractions from more serious preterm labor. Today, we have two tools to help make that distinction: *fetal fibronectin* and *salivary estriol testing*. Fetal fibronectin is found in fetal membranes; normally, between 24 and 36 weeks, levels are undetectable or very low in cervical secretions, but increase with labor. If the fetal fibronectin level is low, there is a 99 percent chance you will not deliver in the next week; a negative fetal fibronectin swab allows you to avoid taking tocolytic drugs. Salivary estriol, a measure of a type of estrogen in your saliva, also increases prior to delivery, whether that delivery happens on time or early. If salivary estriol levels increase, then risk of preterm delivery is higher, and tocolysis can be begun.

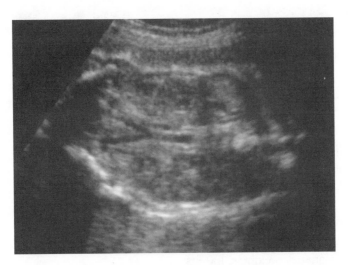

"A fork in the road. This ultrasound shows the branching of the aorta, the large artery that takes blood from the heart to the rest of the body, dividing into the right and left iliac arteries (supplying the lower body)."

Some women are more likely to experience preterm labor than others. The biggest contributing factors are carrying twins or more, history of a previous preterm delivery, and lack of prenatal care. Infection, particularly *bacterial vaginosis,* may increase the risk of preterm labor. If you have had a preterm delivery in a previous pregnancy, the risk of recurrence ranges from 17 to 37 percent. Other risk factors are listed in table 30.1. Age, as you may be happy to hear, is not as big a factor as some of the others, and you may notice that the under-18 crowd is also at risk.

Because complications from preterm delivery are so costly, both on a personal level and on a national, economic level, there have been many attempts to prevent preterm labor and delivery. Ranging

TABLE 30.1

Risk Factors for Preterm Labor

Abnormalities of the uterus (bicornuate uterus, T-shaped uterus, fibroids)

Age < 18 or > 40

Alcohol abuse

Cigarette smoking

Fetal abnormalities

Greater than three previous first-trimester miscarriages or abortions, or one second-trimester

Multiple gestation

Illegal drug use

Incompetent cervix

Infection

No prenatal care

Pre-pregnancy weight < 100 lbs.

Prior preterm delivery

from frequent doctor visits and cervical exams to home uterine activity monitoring for women with risk factors, none have been found to be terribly effective on a global level—for individual women, sure, but not on a national scale. Frequent telephone contact with a specially trained nurse has been found to be as effective in preventing preterm birth as high-tech—and much more expensive—home monitoring. Reduced activity and increasing bed rest is another approach to preventing preterm births. Again, there are no clear-cut studies showing statistically significant benefit; however, it doesn't hurt, and I can guarantee if you are having preterm labor your doctor is going to tell you to take it easy.

Signs of preterm labor are regular contractions, often more frequent and more intense than the Braxton Hicks contractions you have been experiencing; increase in vaginal discharge; increase in pelvic pressure; low backache, especially if it is rhythmic; diarrhea; and spotting, especially if accompanied by any of the other symptoms. If you experience any of these, contact your doctor. Do not worry about bothering your doctor—you are paying her for this!

If you think you are having preterm labor, you will be instructed to go either to the office or the hospital for monitoring and an exam. If you are indeed in preterm labor (remember, you have to be contracting and your cervix has to be either dilated or *effaced*), you will be given medication to stop the contractions; what you are given depends on how much you are dilated and how much you are contracting. The only FDA-approved tocolytic is *ritodrine;* however, it is the least commonly used. Most medications used to treat preterm labor are used "off label," meaning that these drugs are FDA approved for other conditions but have been found to be effective in halting preterm labor as well. *Magnesium sulfate* is the most commonly used IV tocolytic, and *terbutaline* (brand name *Brethine*), which can be given by subcutaneous (just under the skin) injection or orally, is the medication the majority of women are sent home on. Table 30.2 lists different classes of tocolytics and the potential side effects associated with them.

TABLE 30.2

Tocolytics and Their Side Effects

Medication	Effects on You	Effects on Baby
Beta-adrenergic agents (ritodrine, terbutaline)	Increased heart rate; low blood pressure; jitteriness; insomnia; impaired glucose tolerance (increased risk of gestational diabetes)	Increased heart rate
Magnesium sulfate	Muscle weakness; nausea; hot flushes; low blood pressure; respiratory depression (if toxic doses given)	Muscle weakness and respiratory depression if delivered during or shortly after magnesium given. Lowers risk the baby will develop intraventricular hemorrhage
Prostaglandin inhibitors (indomethacin)	Stomach upset; GI bleeding; Premature closure of the ductus arteriosis; decreased amniotic fluid volume; intraventricular hemorrhage	
Calcium channel blocker (nifedipine)	Low blood pressure	

If you have to be hospitalized for preterm labor and are given magnesium sulfate, you will probably also receive a shot of a steroid, usually *betamethasone*, to help your baby's lungs mature faster. Steroids have also been shown to decrease the chance the baby might have an *intraventricular hemorrhage* (IVH; see week 24). The effect of steroids is temporary, so if you get through one bout of preterm labor, only to be readmitted 10 days later, the dose of steroids will need to be repeated. If you do deliver early, steroids can make the difference between your baby developing respiratory distress or not. Antibiotics are also frequently given to women experiencing preterm labor for two reasons: infection is a possible cause of preterm labor, and premature babies are more likely to be adversely affected if you are carrying the *Group B Strep* (GBS) bacteria. Antibiotics given in labor can decrease the odds of your baby becoming very ill from GBS.

Experts today recommend treating each acute episode of preterm labor with a course of tocolytics to stop the contractions and allow time to administer the steroids. If the contractions stop easily, they recommend you not be maintained on an oral tocolytic. If you experience another bout of preterm labor, you would be treated again, only until that episode was resolved. Most doctors practicing in the "real world," outside the confines of an academic center, are probably still sending moms home on terbutaline and bed rest until the thirty-seventh week; old habits are hard to break, even if they are not supported by scientific evidence.

Frequently Asked Questions

Q I delivered my first child at 34 weeks, and am already 1 cm dilated at 30 weeks with number two. My doctor has told me to practice pelvic rest and to stay off my feet. I'm having no problems with the first directive, but how am I supposed to be at bed rest when I have a 3-year-old son?

A *Bed rest can be a hard instruction to follow. First, get exact, explicit instructions on exactly what you can and cannot do—can you get up to take a shower and eat meals, or must you be confined to bed all day and all night, using a commode placed at the bedside? The latter is often called* strict bed rest, *while a bit more freedom is called* modified bed rest. *Second, get help—from spouse, family, and friends. Even if you are allowed to get up a little, don't waste your time or energy cooking or cleaning; delegate those tasks to someone else.*

As for mothering a toddler while confined to the bed or couch, there are tasks that you can delegate. If you don't want to send your toddler off to day care all day, have a teenager come after school to play with your child while you rest. Explain to your little one that you have to stay quiet, and you would love to read to him, watch videos, and play quiet games, all of which you can do while reclining. Toddlers understand a heck of a lot more than we adults give them credit for, and they aim to please. Rent or borrow a small refrigerator and keep it near you, stocked with snacks for you and your child—a 3-year-old can open the door and get his sippy cup of milk (left there by one of your helpers every morning!) and bring you an apple. He will be happy to be near you—and very pleased that he can help you.

Q **I have been having contractions for several weeks. They aren't Braxton Hicks because they are strong and regular. I keep going in for checks, but my cervix is still long and closed. The doctor put me on terbutaline but the side effects are awful. Is there any way I can stop taking it?**

A *Do not stop taking the terbutaline—or any other prescribed medication—without talking to your doctor first. You can ask your doctor about doing one of the newer tests to assess your risk of early delivery. One protocol suggests doing a fetal fibronectin swab; if the result is negative, a salivary estriol is done. If that is also negative, your chances of delivering prematurely are exceedingly low, and you may stop the terbutaline. Your cervix is checked weekly to make sure it is not opening, and the salivary estriol is repeated every 2 weeks. I recently managed a patient this way—she had been placed on terbutaline for preterm contractions that occurred while traveling to another state. When she returned home I did a fetal fibronectin (negative) and stopped her terbutaline. Despite continuing contractions, every-other-week salivary estriol tests were also negative. Her due date is next week, and we never did have to use terbutaline again. Now she's trying every trick in the book to make labor happen!*

Q My membranes ruptured yesterday, at 31 weeks. The doctors have me on magnesium sulfate in order to allow time to give me two steroid shots. I'm also on antibiotics. They say after today they are going to stop the magnesium and follow "expectant management." What does that mean?

A *Premature rupture of the membranes (PROM) is a factor in 25 to 33 percent of all premature births. Because steroids can significantly reduce the risk of respiratory distress in your baby, they are administered unless you show signs of infection. If there is evidence of infection (fever, uterine tenderness, foul vaginal discharge, fetal distress), the baby is delivered. However, if the baby appears to be doing well and there is no sign of infection, the tocolytics are stopped but antibiotics are continued for 7 days (IV for the first two days, then orally). You will probably stay in the hospital, where you and the baby can be monitored closely. Daily non-stress tests (NSTs) are done—see week 35 to learn more about* antenatal testing. *If at any point you develop an infection or your baby shows any signs of compromise (as evidenced by "flunking" an antenatal test), your labor will be induced. Otherwise,* expectant management *means watching and waiting until you go into labor on your own; 75 percent of women with PROM will deliver within 1 week.*

Week 31

SUN _____ DATE _____

MON _____ DATE _____

TUE _____ DATE _____

WED _____ DATE _____

THUR _____ DATE _____

FRI _____ DATE _____

SAT _____ DATE _____

What Happened This Week?

_____

_____

_____

_____

How I Feel Physically and Emotionally

_____

_____

_____

_____

It's a Family Affair

You HAVE A husband, a mate, a partner. You have other children, perhaps a blended family—his kids, your kids, and a new one on the way. You have a mother and father and in-laws. You may be doing this solo, but you have family and friends who love you and are there to support you. You may be the one carrying the baby, but those around you are "with child" too. This week's Special Considerations is for them.

What Baby Is Doing

Your baby continues to plump up, looking more like the Gerber baby every day. The delicate tracings of blood vessels are no longer visible under her skin. She is perfecting skills she will need after birth, like sucking. Her urinary system is working quite well, and part of the amniotic fluid is urine your baby has passed. This once again is practice: It is estimated a baby will soil about 2,500 diapers from birth until she is fully toilet trained!

Your little one is 27.5 cm (11 in) sitting and a hair under 39 cm (15.5 in) standing. She weighs 1,500 gm (3 lbs. 5 oz.).

What You Are Doing

Your uterus pretty much fills your abdominal cavity now, from pubic bone to rib cage. You may feel as if your baby's feet are stuck under your ribs. You may also notice some discomfort under the right side of your rib cage, especially after eating a fatty meal. This could reflect gallbladder disease. Thanks to high estrogen levels during pregnancy, gallstones are more likely to form. Gallbladder disease is also more common in women over 40.

WHAT DADS HAVE TO SAY

I asked several of my over-35-year-old patients' significant others how they coped with mom-to-be's hormonal upheavals.

Rick, age 37, and about to be a first-time dad: "Pathetically, I mean sympathetically! I was definitely sensitive and aware and helped out as much as I could."

Jeff, my husband: "What hormonal moodiness? You were your usual wonderful self." I must note this was accompanied by a drawing of me holding a gun to his head and saying "be nice!"

David, age 37: "She really hasn't changed at all. The pregnancy has been great—no morning sickness, just a little backache now, but she doesn't complain about it."

Karl, age 44, father to a 5-year-old: "Tolerance, lots of tolerance."

Special Considerations

FOR DADS-TO-BE

Dads or non-pregnant partners often feel like old shoes, left out of all the attention and excitement. Remember, it takes both an egg and a sperm to make a baby, and although you may not be the one with the bulging belly (or maybe your belly is growing too!), you are still involved and incredibly important. I really like the phrase "We're pregnant" to convey that it does take more than just Mom to have a healthy baby. I love it when dads come to the prenatal visits and I can see the look of awe in your eyes when you hear your baby's heartbeat for the very first time. No, you cannot share the morning sickness and the hemorrhoids, but you can help in many, many other ways. You can do the laundry and grocery shopping in the first trimester, when your mate is nauseous and exhausted. You can take her out to dinner in the second trimester, just to celebrate how wonderful she looks pregnant. You can show an interest in picking out all the baby accoutrements (if you really could care less about Winnie the Pooh versus clowns, fake it!).

You may be the most interested parent-to-be in the world, but Mom-to-be is making all the decisions without you. Speak up. She is not perfect, and she may assume you won't care about details or that you don't want to know about the backache she has every day. We women secretly wish men were psychic, and we don't want to have to tell you what we want; we just want you to know it. That is our little quirk, and you can help avoid being on the receiving end of a hormonally driven emotional outburst by (1) letting us know you want to be involved, and (2) asking us simply, "What's new?" or "What can I do for you today?" I assumed my husband wouldn't care how I decorated the nursery, and I was pleasantly surprised when he gave his opinion (we eventually agreed on Winnie the Pooh). Certainly, you should be involved in all medical decisions regarding your baby, especially in deciding on genetic testing. It may be her body, and I do believe the ultimate decision is hers, but it is your baby too, and you should have input.

Don't worry if it takes you a while to bond with your developing baby. Some men fall in love as soon as the pregnancy test is positive, but most have to hold their baby for bonding to take place. Often, the pregnancy may not seem completely real to you until after your mate begins to show or after you can feel the baby kick through her belly. You may be worried that something might go wrong, and you don't want to get too attached too soon. You may be worried about your wife; when she is in the bathroom retching every morning, it is easy to think it's your fault she's so miserable. You may be worried about whether you'll be a good father, if this is your first, or whether you can love this baby as much as your others, if you are a veteran. She may not tell you, but, believe me, she is wondering the same thing about herself. If you share your feelings with her, both your fears and your joys, you will become closer and will enjoy each other and this pregnancy that much more.

Another way you can both be supportive and involved is to attend childbirth classes. You may feel silly sitting on the floor with a bunch of twentysomethings, but that will soon pass. Even if you already have children, especially if this is the first baby the two of you are having together, I encourage you to go to the classes. Read this and other books together. Make a list of possible names; my husband came up with some doozies, and he'd always throw out a particularly outrageous one when I needed a good laugh. Share the good and the bad. If she has to quit smoking, you should too, not only to make it easier on her, but to make your baby healthier. She's not drinking, so you can cut down as well—at least wait to open that Screaming Eagle until she can enjoy a glass as well! If she's having fruit for dessert, you can just put away that box of double fudge cookies, thank you.

Enjoy the experience of being a pregnant couple. Be involved. Talk to your growing baby throughout the weeks and months, and when you whisper his name and pick him up for the first time, and he stops crying and stares into your face with a puzzled expression, then you will know you are a dad.

FOR OTHER CHILDREN

Obviously, your 2-year-old is not going to be able to read this himself, so I'll direct this to you adults. You may wonder how you are going to be able to nurture this developing baby when you have a toddler clinging to your leg all the time. You may wonder how you can possibly love this baby as much as you do your first. Love

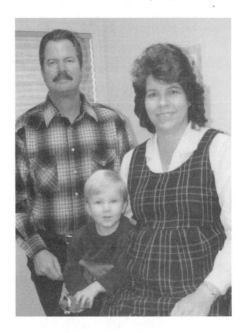

"Family affair. Michelle, age 39; husband, Steve; and son, Daniel; all participate in prenatal visits."

has a way of expanding, so there is always plenty to go around. Yes, life as your toddler knows it is about to change, but change is often for the good. A toddler thinks he is center of the universe, and moving him gently from being the sole object of your attention can help a toddler mature. If you have to throw up when your little one wants a book read *now,* he will learn patience and to wait his turn. If you just cannot get up from the couch because you are so exhausted, he will learn to help you. If you cannot run and pick him up every time he stumbles, he may learn to soothe himself. This is not an easy task, but the whole family will benefit from it.

Little children have no sense of time. A younger-than-2-year-old is not going to understand the concept of a baby growing in you in the first place, and certainly is not going to understand that her new little brother or sister is not going to arrive for several more months. It is best to wait to tell the news until you are very pregnant—about 34–36 weeks. You can then talk about the new baby who is going to arrive, showing your child pictures of newborns. You can bring your toddler to a prenatal visit to listen to the baby's heartbeat. A preschooler can be told a little earlier, maybe as soon as you are obviously pregnant, but again, their attention span is pretty short. Preschoolers love to help Mommy, and being pregnant when your older child is in the 4 to 5 range is especially rewarding (from what I've heard, being the mother of just one child myself!).

You may be thinking about including your older children in the delivery. I don't think the delivery room is appropriate for a child much under the age of 4—seeing you in pain, seeing the blood and the mess is probably way more than the average toddler can handle. It is best for young toddlers to stay home with a trusted and familiar caregiver, and go visit Mom and new baby in the hospital after everything has settled down. Preschoolers and older children may relish the experience of seeing their younger sibling being born, and may feel a special bond because they witnessed the birth. Special sibling classes or videos can be helpful in preparing your older children for what they will see and hear. You as the parent know the temperament of your child best; not all children will do well seeing Mommy in pain or complying with the need to be relatively quiet and not run amok all over the labor and delivery ward. You should always arrange for the help of a familiar person whose focus can be on your older child and who can allow you to focus on the birth of the new baby.

Older children often feel as left out as Dad. One way to help circumvent this is for you—and family and friends—to include the other children. Of course everyone will want to know how you are doing during the pregnancy, but they can also ask Junior if he's felt his new baby brother move yet. T-shirts can proudly proclaim, "I'm the big brother!" One couple I delivered (actually, I delivered both their sons) had planned ahead: when the two-and-a-half-year-old came in with a stuffed animal for his new baby brother, there was a gift all wrapped up in colorful paper from the new baby to him. It helped him feel special and bonded to "my wittle brudder."

FOR FAMILY AND FRIENDS

I'll keep my advice to you short and sweet. Don't tell horror stories about your pregnancy or birth. Don't tell your daughter-in-law (or daughter, for that matter), "Oh my goodness, you'll hurt my grandchild if you go to the gym; sit on the couch right now, young lady!" Don't criticize her looks, her clothes, or the fact that she is planning on returning to work when the baby is 6 weeks old. Do tell her— both of them—that you love them, you are thrilled they are having a baby (even if you secretly think they are nuts for having another child; three is enough already and besides, she's almost 40!), and you will do whatever you can to help. And then do it. Bring over casseroles to keep in the freezer. Take older children to the park so Mom can get a pedicure. Give Mom a gift certificate for a massage. Be loving, not smothering; supportive, not critical.

Frequently Asked Questions

Q This is going to be the first grandchild on either side of the family. My mother took to wearing black, mourning the fact she'd never be a grandmother, until I surprised her by marrying my husband at age 38 and promptly getting pregnant! She wants to be here for the delivery, and so do my in-laws, delightful people who drive me nuts under the best of circumstances. When my mother and mother-in-law get together . . . What can I do? I do not want my baby's birth to be a 3-ring circus.

A *Oh yes, the grandparent dilemma. You love them, they love you, but you really want your birthing experience to be a special moment for you and your husband alone. I had the same dilemma. I am an only child, my widowed mother lives 3,000 miles away, and*

I'm finally about to give her the grandchild she's been hoping for ever since I said, "I do," but I only want Jeff in the delivery room, and we both want to get used to this whole parenthood thing on our own first. Fortunately, my mom spared me the agony of telling her this—she called one day and said she hoped I didn't want her at the birth because she thought it should be a private time between Jeff and me. My mom is a great woman (exasperating at times, but great nonetheless!)—I know you were lying, Mom, and you would have given your right arm to have been there for Hunter's birth, and I love you for it!

If your mother and mother-in-law don't let you off the hook so easily (you could try leaving this book sitting around, opened to this page), you and your husband will have to tell them. You tell your mom and let him tell his. Tell them you know how excited they are, but you really want this to be a quiet, special moment for the two of you. Tell them they can really help out by washing all the baby's new clothes and feeding the dogs while you do all that nasty, sweaty labor stuff. Tell them you couldn't possibly focus on pushing if they were in the room, you are just too modest. ("Remember, Mom, you haven't seen me naked since I was 7" might work.) And when all else fails, tell them it's hospital policy that only one person can be in the labor room, and heck, Mom, I know you gave birth to me, but my husband (wife) will be so upset if I tell him (her) I picked you instead!

Q I've been having a sharp pain on my right side for weeks, and it is getting worse. It usually happens after I eat, and last night after pepperoni pizza it was awful. My mom says it is my gallbladder and I'm going to have to have surgery.

A *You mom is probably right—at least halfway. Pain high on the right side, under the ribcage, may be from gallstones. Thanks to high hormone levels, a pregnant woman is more likely to develop gallstones, which can cause pain. You may not need surgery, however. Because the gallbladder has to work harder to help you digest a fatty meal, gallbladder pain may be more pronounced after a greasy pizza. By watching your diet and avoiding greasy, fatty, or heavy foods, you may be able to control your symptoms without the need for the gall-bladder to be removed. Gallstones usually do not dissolve by themselves, so surgery is a possibility in the future; it is easier to do and there are no worries about baby if it is delayed until after you deliver.*

Week 32

SUN	DATE
MON	DATE
TUE	DATE
WED	DATE
THUR	DATE
FRI	DATE
SAT	DATE

What Happened This Week?

How I Feel Physically and Emotionally

Learning About Labor

M ORE AND MORE couples take childbirth education classes, and even if you have had children before, a refresher class is a good idea. In our mothers' day, women were heavily medicated and fathers were banished to the waiting room, so learning about labor was a non-issue. Today, we want more information about what to expect in the delivery room.

What Baby Is Doing

Your baby's nervous system matures each and every day. Beginning this week, the pupils will constrict if a bright light is shone in the baby's face. The surface of the brain is becoming more and more convoluted as the brain grows. This folding of brain tissue allows us to have large brains, capable of thinking great thoughts, innovating, and basically doing all the things that make us human, without having heads the size of watermelons.

Your baby's brain and head are continuing to grow, but not as rapidly as the rest of the body. The head is now more proportional to the body. The skull is not a solid helmet, but rather is a series of bones, joined together by flexible membranous *sutures* that allow the baby's head to mold to fit through the birth canal and allow for continued brain growth after birth. If these sutures close too soon, the head can be misshapen.

Your baby now weighs 1,700 gm (3 lbs. 11 oz.). Crown–rump length is 28 cm (11.2 in) and total length is 40 cm (16 in).

What You Are Doing

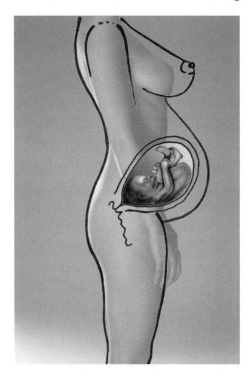

At 32 weeks, you have a noticeable swayback from your ever-expanding uterus. Your baby may decide to keep his feet tucked under your ribs, too.

You are probably beginning to think a lot about actually delivering your baby, and may begin to have fears about this whole labor thing. Unless you've been living in a cave, complete strangers have probably come up to you in the grocery store to regale you with unwanted horror stories about their Aunt Mabel's best friend's sister's birth, and to tell you you are too big/too small/shouldn't be carrying that grocery bag. Ignore these people the best you can.

If you have not been troubled by hemorrhoids so far, you may start to notice them. Caused by the pressure of your by-now quite large uterus (32 cm—almost 13 inches—from your pubic bone!), they afflict a large percentage of pregnant women. The good news is they will be less troublesome after you deliver, but the bad news is they probably won't go away completely.

Special Considerations

You obviously want to learn about pregnancy, your unborn child, and how to cope with your labor and delivery, or else you wouldn't be reading this book. You are probably planning to take some type of prepared childbirth class. If you are not, I'd encourage you to rethink that decision. A good childbirth education class can mentally, physically, and emotionally prepare you for the rigors of giving birth. Even if you have had children before, consider a refresher class, especially if you and your spouse have not had a child together. I'm an obstetrician and I took a class! As I told my patients who were in the class with me, I had never given birth myself, my

husband had never had a child, he wasn't in the medical field, and we just wanted to experience what everyone else does.

One of the biggest benefits to taking a childbirth class is learning about what you will see, feel, and hear while in the labor and delivery suite. I firmly believe that the more you know, the less you fear, and the less you fear, the less pain you will have. Knowledge is power, the power to conquer the fear of the unknown.

Different types of childbirth education classes emphasize different things, but most give you an overview of the process, from checking in, to getting (or not) an IV, to the stages of labor and the delivery itself, and teach some technique to help you relax

From My Journal
"The childbirth classes are okay. Obviously, I know most of what is taught, but having Jeff hear it and just us doing this together as a couple—preparing to be a family—is worthwhile. Sometimes I wish I had gone off the hill, where nobody knows I'm an ob-gyn, so I could just be another mom-to-be instead of half the class's doctor."

during your labor. The three most common philosophies are Grantly Dick-Read, Lamaze, and Bradley, although most classes offered by a hospital, birthing center, or through your doctor's office will be a bit of this and a bit of that, often with more of an emphasis on process rather than relaxation. Grantly Dick-Read was an English obstetrician, the author of *Childbirth Without Fear*. His philosophy forms the cornerstone of all methods taught today, although Dr. Dick-Read felt that if medication could help break the fear-pain cycle then it should be used liberally. Lamaze is the most popular method, introduced by French obstetrician Dr. Fernand Lamaze. The key to Lamaze is learning breathing patterns to distract you from the pain of labor. Your husband-coach reminds you to breath away your pain. Lamaze also teaches the advantages and disadvantages of medical options for pain control (which will be discussed in detail in week 38), but encourages avoiding routine medical intervention. The Bradley Method, developed in the 1940s by U.S. obstetrician Dr. Robert Bradley, introduced the concept of using the husband as coach. Its philosophy centers on experiencing and accepting the pain, and not using artificial methods (specific breathing patterns, drugs, epidurals) to mask or escape it; there is a definite emphasis on unmedicated labor. Changing body positions to what works best for you and doing deep abdominal breathing are taught, but at its most basic, Bradley teaches you to trust yourself. In table 32.1 you will find contact information for various childbirth education groups.

If you live where I do, there isn't much choice in childbirth education—there's the class offered by the hospital and taught by one of the labor and delivery nurses. These classes can be excellent, as mine was, and an advantage is that the person teaching the class works where you will deliver and knows exactly what the logistics are, and also has worked with the doctor who will be doing your delivery. The disadvantage is that if you are really interested in learning about a particular method, like Bradley, you are out of luck. If you live in a larger community, you may have several alternatives: Lamaze, a Bradley instructor, a private one-on-one teacher, in addition to classes sponsored by the local hospital or your insurance company.

I am all for a "natural" childbirth, but I have a problem with teachers who suggest, however subtly, that you are a failure if you choose an epidural or end up with a cesarean section. There are no failures when it comes to having a baby—no matter what it takes to get there, the only goal should be to hold a healthy baby in your arms. If you can do that by relying on your inner strength, that is wonderful, but if you need or choose medical intervention, that is great, too—it is your birth experience, after all, not the childbirth education instructor's.

Because fear of the unknown can contribute to anxiety and pain, I do encourage you to take a class sponsored by your doctor or the hospital where you will deliver. These classes usually spend a fair amount of time discussing what I call process issues: where to go when you are admitted; hospital (or your own doctor's) policy on fetal monitoring; use of IVs; what the various fetal monitoring devices look like and when they are likely to be used; mechanism of labor and delivery itself; what will happen if you need a cesarean section. They often include a tour of the facility, so you will have an opportunity to see where you are going to have your baby. By learning the particulars of your hospital, there will be less to be afraid of when you walk in the doors in labor.

While hospital-based classes do discuss relaxation techniques, if available, I would also encourage you to take a Bradley or Lamaze or other "natural" childbirth class. These classes can help you realize the power you have within you, potent knowledge not only in the delivery room, but also in the weeks, months, and years of childraising ahead of you. But, please, if you do take one of these classes, do not think you will be a failure if what you learn is not enough and you choose to take medication or an epidural.

TABLE 32.1

Childbirth Education Resources

The Bradley Method
American Academy of Husband-Coached Childbirth
Box 5224
Sherman Oaks, CA 91413-5224
1 800-4 A BIRTH
www.bradleybirth.com

International Childbirth Education Association
P.O. Box 20038
Minneapolis, MN 55420
612-854-8600

Doulas of North America (DONA)
13513 North Grove Avenue
Alpine, UT 84004
801-756-7331
www.dona.com

Lamaze International
2025 M Street NW, Suite 800
Washington, DC 20036-3309
800-368-4404
www.lamaze-childbirth.com

While not strictly childbirth education, another option is to hire a doula to assist you in labor and to attend the childbirth classes with you and your partner. *Doula* is Greek for "woman's servant," and she is trained in providing emotional and physical support to you during your labor. She will help you get as comfortable as possible and will support you in whatever choices you make during your labor. A doula is a complement to your husband or significant other, not a replacement, allowing that person to concentrate more on the experience and worry less about running out to get you ice chips.

Frequently Asked Questions

Q I live in a big city, and there are a zillion options for childbirth classes. Are there any criteria I can use to decide which are good and which are not?

A *First, ask your doctor for a recommendation. This will help minimize conflict between your doctor's philosophy and that of the instructor; of course, you may be looking for a different viewpoint in the first place, in which case, ignore this advice! If any questions arise in class, be sure to talk them over with your doctor. (You did evaluate your doctor's style of practice before you chose her, right?)*

Second, look for a relatively small class of no more than 10 couples—five to six is ideal. In addition to learning about labor, one of the benefits of taking a prenatal class is the camaraderie that develops, and this is more easily accomplished in a smaller group. Third, get an outline of what will be covered, making sure it includes the physiology of labor, as well as all options for pain control, even if the emphasis is on an unmedicated birth. In order to convey all the information needed, most good classes last at least 6 weeks. Ask if there is give-and-take, or if the class is conducted as a lecture.

Finally, talk to other women who have given birth recently and ask them about the classes they took. Find out what they liked—and disliked—about the class and instructor, and whether the information helped them during labor.

Q My mother just had surgery for hemorrhoids, a miserable experience that she blames on her six children. Am I destined to have the same fate, or is there something I can do to prevent hemorrhoids?

A *Painful, itchy, bleeding hemorrhoids are not inevitable. While you cannot do anything about the physiology that contributes to them (big uterus compressing the vena cava and increasing pressure downstream), you can take steps to minimize problems. The most important thing to do is to avoid constipation; if you have to strain to have a bowel movement, you will put even more pressure on those veins around your rectum, causing hemorrhoids to pop out. Drink lots of water (at least six to eight 8-ounce glasses a day), and increase fiber, too. If you eat a lot of fiber and don't drink enough fluids, you can actually worsen constipation. Regular exercise also keeps the bowels regular and decreases constipation. Avoid laying flat on your back; by staying on one side or the other, you will keep the bulk of your uterus off the vena cava and decrease the pressure build up in the rectal veins.*

If, despite all your best efforts, hemorrhoids do flare up, you can use over-the-counter preparations to ease the discomfort. Very, very rarely, if a hemorrhoid clots off (medical term is thromboses*), it may need to be lanced to alleviate the exceedingly painful pressure.*

Q I've just started to notice a sharp pain running from my bottom and down the back of my right leg. What is this, and more importantly, what do I do about it?

A *You are describing sciatica, another consequence of that enlarging uterus. In this case, your uterus—or the baby's head as it* snuggles into place—is putting pressure on the sciatic nerve, the longest nerve in the human body. The pain, usually stabbing in nature, can be excruciating, but it usually comes and goes in response to position changes. Gentle stretching exercises and avoiding postures that exacerbate the pain are the best means of prevention. While sleeping, lie on your side with a pillow between your knees. When standing, alternate propping one foot then the other on a low box or stool. The best stretches for sciatica are:

Tailor Sitting. Sit on the floor with knees bent and soles of your feet together. You can gently press down on your knees to give a bit more stretch. Stay in this position for 5–10 minutes a couple of times a day.

Pelvic Tilt. Stand against a wall, pressing your lower back into the wall and then relaxing. Repeat this several times.

Dromedary Droop. Get on the floor on your hands and knees. Roll your back up, like a camel's hump, and look down. Then relax and let your back drop down as you look up.

Week 33

SUN _____ DATE _____

MON _____ DATE _____

TUE _____ DATE _____

WED _____ DATE _____

THUR _____ DATE _____

FRI _____ DATE _____

SAT _____ DATE _____

What Happened This Week?

_____

_____

_____

How I Feel Physically and Emotionally

_____

_____

_____

Blueprint for Birth

BIRTH PLANS SEEM to be the hot things to write as the twenty-first century begins—nary a day goes by without a very pregnant woman bringing hers in for me to review. While most are pretty sensible, they do need to be flexible. My husband is a builder, and he is supposed to follow a blueprint when building a house (or my new office building!), but I know a window is moved here and a door a few inches there once the real work begins; you have to make adjustments when the living room window on the blueprint looks directly into the bedroom of the real-life house next door—or when those breathing exercises just aren't enough for the pain of labor.

What Baby Is Doing

Your baby's fingernails have reached the ends of her fingers, and her toenails are not far behind. She still has a fair amount of room in which to move, so her kicks and punches can be quite forceful. Space is getting tighter, however, so the somersaults of weeks past are at an end. She does have enough room to turn around if she happens to be breech now, but if she doesn't find her way to being head first soon, she is unlikely to do so on her own.

At 33 weeks, your baby is 41 cm tall (about 16½ in); the crown–rump length is 29 cm (11½ in). Your baby has broken the 4-pound barrier—weight is now 1,900 gm, or 4 lbs. 3 oz.

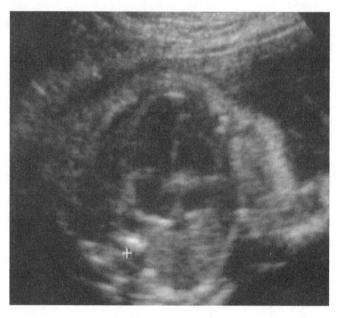

"And the beat goes on. . . .This ultrasound of the heart shows all four chambers in cross section."

What You Are Doing

You may have discovered it is more difficult to find a comfortable sleeping position. Your expanding uterus (now 33 ± 2 cm from the top of your pubic bone) is crowding your lungs; you may find you have less shortness of breath if you sleep propped up. Many a pregnant woman spends the night in the La-Z-Boy at this point! If you are able to stay in bed, be sure to sleep on one side or the other, and never flat on your back. A body pillow can be a great help in positioning you comfortably. I used two body pillows when I was pregnant, with my upper leg resting on one in front, and one in back to keep me from accidentally rolling over. My husband didn't really like them, as they kept him from snuggling as close—in fact, I think he hid them as soon as Hunter moved from our bed to her crib!

Special Considerations

A good birth plan outlines your preferences as to what your labor, delivery, and immediate postpartum experience will be like; it is realistic and flexible. A birth plan is a wish list; it is not a contract written in stone. You have probably already talked over your preferences with your doctor, but a written birth plan will allow your preferences to be known by the nursing staff, your support people,

✎ DOCTOR'S NOTES

Here was my birth plan: "Deliver Hunter." It's probably a bit too short, unless you are an obstetrician being delivered by one of your own associates, in the hospital in which you practice, and attended by a nurse of your own choosing!

I have seen many a woman have a bad experience because her plan was so inflexible. One woman was adamant she have an epidural—it was written in all caps, bold, and underlined in her birth plan. Well, she got to the hospital and was 9 cm dilated, and delivered 30 minutes later. She could not get beyond the fact that she didn't get an epidural. She couldn't see how lucky she was that she only had to push three times to deliver an 8-pound, beautiful, healthy baby (her first, by the way) and not even have an episiotomy or a tear.

and a covering doctor if your own doc is not available. Do you have to write a birth plan? Heck no! But, it can be a useful tool to get you and your partner thinking about the type of experience you hope your baby's birth will be. Also, in today's climate of managed care and short office visits, it gives everyone an opportunity to make sure all your concerns and hopes are addressed.

Flexibility is the key word in birth plans. All of us—doctors, midwives, nurses, you, your spouse, family, and friends—want you to have a great birth. If you are rigid and demanding, however, you will alienate your medical team and will be doomed to failure. Your doctor and the nursing staff need to be flexible, too. If your doctor cuts an episiotomy every time, "just because," and you wish to avoid an episiotomy, this needs to be discussed ahead of time. Your doctor should be able to grant you this wish.

A good birth plan is no more than one page long, clear and concise. This is not the place to hone your creative writing skills. Your doctor is pressed for time, the nurses at the hospital are pressed for time, and they are not going to struggle through a lot of verbiage. Make your wishes easy to see, at a glance. It is also more productive to be positive in expressing your wishes—use "I'd like" rather than "Don't you dare" phrases. And, you really do not need to put a line in that you don't want an enema and don't want your *perineum* shaved. I started my medical school in 1983; I have delivered babies in eight hospitals in three states and I have never seen an enema given or a perineum shaved for a delivery! And another pretty useless sentence in birth plans I've seen over the years is, "I don't want a cesarean section unless it is absolutely necessary." Guess what? Your doctor doesn't want to do one unless it's necessary either!

A few things you should think about are, Who do you want in the labor room? What kind of "mood" or ambiance do you want? Do you want to bring your own music? How do you feel about an IV? Do you want drugs ASAP or are you trying for an unmedicated birth? What are your feelings about an episiotomy? Do you want Dad to cut the cord? Do you want to hold your baby right away? Do you want the baby to room in? Are you planning to breastfeed or bottlefeed?

Here is a sample birth plan. You can use it as a starting point. Check off those items that appeal to you.

Birth Plan Outline

Name _____

Doctor's name _____

Coach's name _____

Delivering at _____

Other support people _____

Labor preferences: (check all that apply)

___Remain mobile

___Assume whatever position is most comfortable at the time

___Intermittent monitoring of the baby

___Avoid internal monitors if possible

___Saline lock IV rather than being hooked up to fluids the whole time

___Eat lightly and drink fluids liberally

___Calm, soothing atmosphere with low-level lighting, candles, aromatherapy, music

___Allow spontaneous rupture of my membranes

___Avoid pitocin

___Massages

___Warm shower or use of labor tub, if available

___Attempt unmedicated labor and birth, but please give me options if I ask

___Any and all drugs, as soon as possible and as much as possible!

___Epidural as soon as possible

Vaginal delivery preferences: (check all that apply)

___Be in the most comfortable and effective position for me

___Use people rather than stirrups to support my legs

___Use a squat bar

___Use a birthing chair, if available

___Perineal massage

___Avoid vacuum or forceps unless medically indicated or I am absolutely exhausted

___Avoid episiotomy. I'd rather have a small tear

___Please cut an episiotomy. I do not want to tear

___Allow the cord to stop pulsating before cutting it

___My partner will cut the cord

___Place the baby on my chest, skin to skin, right away

In case I need a c-section, my preferences are: (check all that apply)

___My partner with me the entire time

___One hand free to touch my baby

___My partner to hold the baby next to me

___My partner to accompany our baby to the nursery

Newborn care preferences: (check all that apply)

___I plan to breastfeed

___I want to breastfeed immediately after the baby is born

___I plan to bottlefeed

___No pacifiers

___No bottles, unless ordered by my baby's doctor for the health of my baby

___Rooming in

___Take the baby to the nursery so I can sleep undisturbed

Frequently Asked Questions

Q I'm afraid if I write a birth plan my doctor will think I'm questioning her judgment.

A *If you did your homework in the beginning, you have chosen a doctor whose philosophy and "style" mesh with your own. If you have been working as a team all these weeks and months, your doc will not take offense at your birth plan—assuming you've followed the tips above. If you've written a confrontational birth plan, full of sentences like, "Do not even offer me pain medication!" and "I will not have any sort of fetal monitoring," then your doctor will probably be put off by your plan and may even wonder why the heck you are seeking her care. However, if you write a list of things you'd like to have in an ideal world—a wish list—and indicate that you understand circumstances may dictate deviation from that ideal, then the birth plan will serve its purpose: a starting point for discussion of how you'd like your labor to go, and how your support people, your doctor, and the nursing staff can help you get there.*

Q I am huge. I already measure 38 cm and I'm only 33 weeks! The doctor has ordered another ultrasound, and I had one with my CVS and again at 20 weeks, so I know it's not twins or inaccurate dates. What else could be making me so big?

A *There are several possibilities for your size being greater than dates (abbreviated S>D). One is diabetes, especially poorly controlled diabetes. If your sugar levels are high, so are the baby's, and the baby may urinate more, producing more amniotic fluid. The baby himself may be big as well. Another is a problem with the baby's ability to swallow, which can lead to increased amniotic fluid. This can be due to a structural problem, like* esophageal atresia *or* duodenal atresia. *It may also occur if the baby is brain damaged and cannot swallow. You may measure big because you have a large* fibroid, *a benign*

✎ DOCTOR'S NOTES

A NOTHER NEAT THING about journals is that they are a snap-shot of how you were at that moment in time, how you felt, what you were thinking. Reading the entries later can remind you of how much you wanted your child when toddlerhood or the teenage years are particularly challenging. You can also get a good laugh out of some of the things you wrote before you knew what you were talking about. Here's an example of the latter from my journal: comments from today are in brackets: "10/23/98. 33 weeks. Jeff and I have been talking a lot about how we want to raise you—I thought I should get some of these down, if only to see how far off we will be!

1. We will never argue in front of you.

2. You will not watch TV; only videos preselected and approved by us. *Sesame Street* and educational programs on PBS or the Discovery channel are okay. [Okay, so we've bent this a bit—*Teletubbies* are on PBS, but Hunter is addicted. And while she does watch *Baby Mozart* and *Baby Shakespeare*, she has also seen every Disney video. Her current favorite video, excluding "LaLa, Po, Tubbies" is "Mouse, mommy, mouse!" a.k.a. *Stuart Little.*]

3. You will not get every toy on Earth—mainly educational toys and books. *No* video games!!! [We're doing great here, but her baby-sitter buys her toys and stuffed animals at every yard sale she passes!]

tumor of the uterus. Fibroids are very common, increasingly so as we get older.

The ultrasound will tell whether you are big because of too much

4. We will include you in most of our activities and will not alter our lives completely. We will take you hiking and biking and camping [did that at 5 months—sleeping on the ground with an infant is not my idea of fun!] and cross-country skiing right away, and hope you'll be downhill skiing or snowboarding yourself by age two or three. [This has been pretty easy, at least the including part. She's been to Mexico twice, the east coast four times, and wine tasting in Napa at least three times; she's been pushed in front of Rollerblades, pulled behind a bike, paddled in a kayak, and carried in frontpacks and backpacks to the tops of waterfalls and mountain lakes; she was bundled up and taken cross-country skiing at 1 week of age.]

5. No McDonalds or other junky fast foods. [If french fries don't count, I'm still good on this one, although I know her dad and baby-sitter have taken her to the Golden Arches!]

6. We will not force you to clean your plate, but we will make you try everything. [And if she doesn't like it she feeds it to one of our three dogs!]

7. No pacifiers! [Actually, stuck with this one for a full year, and then relented when she started resisting naps. I just "broke" her pacifier by cutting off the nipple, and so far, she's taking it well.]"

Ah, the best laid plans . . .

amniotic fluid, a bigger than expected baby, or something going on with your uterus. Once the "what" is determined, the "why" is sought, especially if the culprit is increased amniotic fluid. If you are so huge *and have so much extra fluid that you are having trouble breathing, an amniocentesis may be necessary periodically to remove the excess fluid until you are delivered.*

Q I can't wait for the baby to be born. I just want to see him now! Is this impatience abnormal?

A *Heck no! There probably isn't a mother in history who hasn't thought, "Enough already, it's about time you were on your own!" It is also normal to want to hold and snuggle and stare at and show off this little being you've been carrying around for months and months already. It is also normal to have the exact opposite feelings (and you may have them tomorrow) of "Don't ever come out, I don't know how to take care of you!" Again, I think it is great to keep a journal of these emotions, so you can share them with your son after he is born. When he is a teenager, you can both look at it and know that, although he may be a pain in the you-know-what now and you can't wait for him to move out of the house, back then you couldn't wait for him to arrive.*

Q My lower back aches so much, especially at the end of the day. What can I do to help relieve the pain and pressure? I don't think I can get through the rest of this pregnancy!

A *Lower backache is one of the most common complaints of the third trimester. Backache occurs because your center of gravity shifts forward as your uterus expands; this causes the characteristic lumbar lordosis, or swayback of pregnancy. Our friend progesterone also plays a role in backache, by relaxing the ligaments and muscles and, therefore, increasing the odds of strain. Good posture goes a long way in relieving lower backache; standing (and sitting) tall, chest out, shoulders back, and pelvis tilted will help keep you from arching your back even more. When picking up objects or other children, bend your legs, keep your back straight, and let your legs do most of the work.*

Massage is a wonderful way to soothe your back—and your psyche. I had a massage every 3–4 weeks during my pregnancy, and I swear it is why I didn't have backaches. (Lord knows it wasn't due to good posture!) Another effective fix for backache is to wear a "belly bra." This is a support sling that cradles your pregnant belly, taking some of the weight and strain off your lower back. There are several varieties available, and they can be found in maternity stores or in ads in the back of pregnancy magazines.

Week 34

SUN _____ DATE

MON _____ DATE

TUE _____ DATE

WED _____ DATE

THUR _____ DATE

FRI _____ DATE

SAT _____ DATE

What Happened This Week?

_____

_____

_____

How I Feel Physically and Emotionally

_____

_____

_____

_____

High Blood Pressure and Pre-Eclampsia

O NCE AGAIN, BEING over 35 places us at increased risk of a complication of pregnancy; in this case, high blood pressure. Chronic, pre-existing high blood pressure is another one of those things that are more common with age. Pre-eclampsia is more common at the extremes of reproductive life, before age 18 and after age 40, and is more common in first-time moms. So, if you develop pre-eclampsia, don't think of yourself as old, think of yourself as "extreme"!

What Baby Is Doing

More and more of the energy-storing white fat is present, accounting for about 8 percent of your baby's total weight. This fat makes the skin now appear pink and smooth; no longer does your baby look like she is wearing clothes two sizes too big.

Your plump little baby weighs 2,100 gm (4 lbs. 9 oz.) and is about 43 cm (17 in) tall. Her crown–rump length is 30 cm (12 in). Despite being bigger than a Cabbage-Patch doll, your baby is still not ready to be born—a lot of maturing will take place in these last 6 weeks.

What You Are Doing

You may not believe it could possibly get any bigger, but your uterus is continuing to grow. At 34 ± 2 cm from your pubic bone, it contains the maximum amount of amniotic fluid at any point in your pregnancy; the volume of your uterus is 500 times greater than it was before you conceived!

In addition to the hemorrhoids we talked about earlier, you may notice varicose veins. Like their hemorrhoid cousins, these dilated veins are caused by the pressure your uterus is placing on all the veins below it.

Special Considerations

Your blood pressure has been checked at each and every one of your prenatal visits. You have been asked to urinate in a cup to see if you are spilling protein. All of this is to catch possible pre-eclampsia early. Pre-eclampsia is a combination of high blood pressure (> 140/90) on at least two readings 6 or more hours apart, coupled with excess protein in the urine (*proteinuria*). Many women will also have more than the usual amount of swelling in the feet, and may have swelling in the hands and face, too. Possible signs of pre-eclampsia are listed in table 34.1. Presence of any of the last four signs listed, or a sensation of just feeling "weird," warrants an immediate call to your doctor, especially if your blood pressure has been elevated. Pre-eclampsia complicates about 6 percent of all pregnancies. Risk factors and their relative chance of causing pre-eclampsia are listed in table 34.2. If you have had pre-eclampsia in a previous pregnancy, your risk of developing it again increases to 7.5 percent. Both a baby aspirin a day and use of high-dose calcium supplements (2,000 mg a day) have shown promise in decreasing the odds of developing pre-eclampsia in high-risk women but talk to your doctor before taking these or any medications.

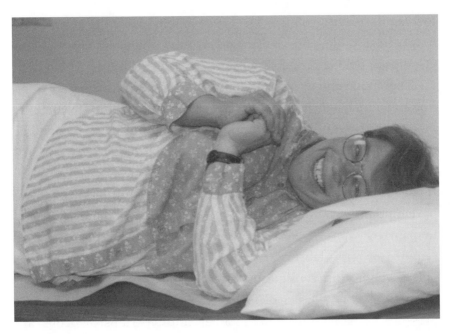

"Bringing down the blood pressure. Marie, age 38, rests on her left side to help lower mildly elevated blood pressure."

Pre-eclampsia is detrimental to both you and your baby. For you, the high blood pressure can impair kidney function. In severe cases, the liver can be affected as well, leading to *HELLP syndrome,* characterized by abnormal liver and blood clotting function. The most serious consequence is progression to *eclampsia.* With eclampsia, seizures occur and a coma may result. In order to save both you and the baby, immediate treatment must be started, and delivery of the baby initiated as soon as you are stable. Eclampsia is extremely uncommon in women who have good prenatal care; your doctor, who is watching you like a hawk, will administer *magnesium sulfate* (discussed following) in order to prevent seizures. I haven't seen a case of eclampsia since I was in my residency.

As far as your baby goes, the high blood pressure of pre-eclampsia increases the risks of placental abruption, growth restriction, and low birthweight, prematurity if early delivery is indicated, and low amniotic fluid volume. The environment inside the uterus is no longer hospitable, and unless you have the mildest of cases of pre-eclampsia, delivery is accomplished.

The management of pre-eclampsia depends on the severity and how far along you are. Mild cases, with only slight elevation in blood pressure and a small amount of protein in the urine, can be managed by bed rest; serial measurements of blood pressure, urinary protein, select blood tests; and fetal monitoring (see week 35). If you are term (37+ weeks) and your cervix is favorable, even if you have mild pre-eclampsia you will likely be induced; there is nothing to gain by waiting. Severe pre-eclampsia or HELLP syndrome requires prompt delivery in order to avoid harm to you and your baby. Magnesium sulfate is started intravenously to prevent seizures; it is not designed to lower blood pressure, and if blood pressure is dangerously high, other antihypertensive drugs are given. Mag sulfate, as it is commonly called, is not pleasant: hot flashes, muscle weakness, headaches, nausea, and drowsiness are common side effects. If you are placed on mag sulfate for seizure prophylaxis (as opposed to treating preterm labor as discussed in week 30), you will also have your bladder continually drained via a Foley catheter. This is necessary to keep close track of how much fluid is going in and how much is coming out, because severe pre-eclampsia can impair kidney function, and too much fluid can lead to *pulmonary edema*. If you and the baby are relatively stable, and there is no sign of fetal distress, a vaginal delivery is usually attempted. If the baby is severely compromised, or if your condition worsens and vaginal delivery is not imminent, a cesarean section is performed.

One of the risk factors for pre-eclampsia and another of the conditions we over-35-year-olds are more likely to have is chronic, pre-existing high blood pressure. High blood pressure decreases blood flow to and through the placenta, resulting in impaired delivery of nutrients and oxygen to your baby, as well as removal of waste products. Poor growth, called IUGR (*intrauterine growth*

TABLE 34.1

Signs of Pre-Eclampsia

High blood pressure, > 140/90 (you won't know this at home)

Proteinuria (again, this is not something you will notice)

Sudden weight gain of > 2 pounds in a week

Excess swelling of the feet, swelling of the hands and face

Headache, not relieved by Tylenol

Pain in the right upper abdomen

Blurry vision

Spots in front of your eyes, especially spots that are stationary

restriction), results, and the baby could possibly be born with a low birthweight. Placental abruption is also a potential consequence of uncontrolled high blood pressure. Unless you develop superimposed pre-eclampsia, pregnancy usually does not increase any risks to you.

If you were hypertensive prior to pregnancy and on medication, you will require medication throughout the pregnancy as well. Some blood pressure medications like ACE inhibitors (Norvasc, Monopril, Accupril, Vasotec, Cozaar are a few examples) are contraindicated during pregnancy and must be changed to a safer antihypertensive. If you were on a beta blocker (Inderal, Tenormin, Normodyne), it usually can be continued. Diuretics may be continued as well, although the baby needs to be closely monitored for normal amniotic fluid volume and proper growth. If you need to be started on a blood pressure medication, or if your current medication needs to be changed, Aldomet (alpha methyldopa) is the first choice in pregnancy. Aldomet has been used since the dawn of time, and its safety and effectiveness in pregnancy is well documented.

Because of the potential for impaired growth of your baby, you

TABLE 34.2

Risk Factors for Pre-Eclampsia

Factor	Relative Risk
Diabetes	2:1
Age > 40	3:1
First pregnancy	3:1
Twins	4:1
Family history of pre-eclampsia	5:1
Chronic hypertension	10:1

will be closely monitored during your pregnancy. Ultrasounds will be done every 3–4 weeks after 20 weeks to make sure your baby is growing. You will start antenatal testing, discussed extensively next week, between 28–32 weeks. You may be asked to see your doctor every 2 weeks starting at 24 weeks in order to make sure you do not show any early signs of superimposed pre-eclampsia. Usually, your pregnancy is not allowed to go much beyond your due date.

Frequently Asked Questions

Q I am 43 and have had high blood pressure for the last 4 years. It's been pretty well controlled on the Normodyne I've taken all along, but on my last ultrasound, the doctor said my baby is developing IUGR. What is that and what do we do about it? It's been a long journey to have this baby, and I don't want anything to happen to her!

A Your doctor doesn't want anything bad to happen to your baby either, which is why your doctor has been getting ultrasounds to monitor the baby's growth. And at this point in the pregnancy, your doctor *has probably already started antenatal testing to check the baby's well-being. IUGR, or intrauterine growth restriction, means the baby is not growing as she should. Usually caused by impaired blood flow through the placenta, a common effect of high blood pressure, it does not allow the baby to get everything she needs to grow. If the baby is noted to fall off the growth curve she has been following, intensive monitoring is begun; the risk is that the baby will become so deprived of oxygen and nutrients that brain damage or even stillbirth could result.*

If the baby's amniotic fluid volume is normal and if antenatal testing is reassuring, you will continue to be monitored. You will probably be placed at modified bed rest in order to ensure as much blood as possible is sent to the placenta (instead of to your muscles, as happens while you are active). You will need to drink lots of fluids and eat properly, and try to avoid stress (yes, I know, you are going to worry about your baby!). Meditation or visualization may help lower blood pressure and improve blood flow to your baby. If all testing remains reassuring and if your baby demonstrates growth from one ultrasound (done every 2–3 weeks now) to the next, you will be allowed to get closer to term. If fluid is extremely low, or if antenatal testing is worrisome, your labor will be induced. If your baby does not tolerate labor, a cesarean section will be necessary.

Q My feet are so swollen. It's August in Dallas and I've been chalking it up to the heat. Now I'm afraid I have pre-eclampsia.

A *Swelling alone does not make pre-eclampsia; if that were the case, every pregnant woman south of the Mason-Dixon line, or on the east coast or the Central Valley of California in the summer would be diagnosed with pre-eclampsia! The diagnosis of pre-eclampsia requires that high blood pressure and excess protein in the urine be present. Not all women with pre-eclampsia, even with severe cases, will have significant swelling. If your swelling has developed rapidly, and if it does not get better by putting your feet up for a few hours, resting on your left side in a cool place, then you should notify your doctor. At home, you are not going to know what your blood pressure is or whether or not you are spilling protein in your urine. Your doctor may have you come in for a quick check just to make sure you have normal Texas summer swelling and are not on the road to pre-eclampsia.*

Q My doctor has diagnosed a mild case of pre-eclampsia and has told me to rest at home, on my side, and to come in twice a week for check ups. I feel fine. I run my own business and really don't want to take the time off if I don't have to.

A *You may feel fine, but if you have pre-eclampsia, you may compromise not only your health but that of your baby by ignoring your doctor's recommendations. Rest helps keep your blood pressure down. Keeping your blood pressure in the normal range helps keep blood, oxygen, and nutrients flowing to your baby. You want your baby to be as healthy as possible, don't you? Well, sometimes that means doing things you don't like to do, like taking it easy and delegating work responsibilities to someone else. You have only one chance to grow a healthy baby; squander it and your baby pays. While work is important, it is not as important as your child.*

Q I could swear my baby is hiccuping. I feel these very rhythmic twitches every so often. Could these really be hiccups?

A *Yes, these could be—and probably are—hiccups. Baby may hiccup after swallowing amniotic fluid. But don't try to yell "Boo" at your belly. Babies can't be scared into stopping like we can!*

Q I've been reading about Group B strep infection. I read that if I have it and pass it on to my baby, my baby could die! When I asked my doctor, she just told me not to worry about it, but I am. How can this infection be prevented?

A Group B streptococcus *(GBS) is a bacteria found in the vagina of 10–30 percent of all pregnant women. It does not cause an infection in these women, and they are usually not even aware they carry the bacteria. GBS can be passed to the baby during delivery. GBS sepsis (blood infection) occurs in newborns in 1.8:1,000 live births; in 6 percent of these cases (or 1:10,000) live births) the baby may die. Most of the time, however, healthy full-term babies do not get sick. Premature babies, with their immature immune systems, are more susceptible. Infection of your baby is also more likely if you have a fever while in labor or if your membranes have been ruptured for more than 18 hours.*

There are two different strategies to prevent GBS infection of newborns, both endorsed by the CDC. The first is to screen all pregnant women by doing a culture of the lower vagina and rectum at 35–37 weeks; if the culture is positive for GBS, you are treated with IV penicillin or a derivative when you go into labor. Treatment is not given before labor, as GBS can return.

The other strategy is to give antibiotics during labor to women with certain risk factors. These risk factors are preterm labor; preterm rupture of membranes; rupture of membranes > 18 hours; previous delivery of a baby with GBS; GBS vaginal or urinary tract infection earlier in the pregnancy; or fever during labor.

There is no evidence that one strategy is better than the other. What is important is that every person delivering babies, and every place in which babies are delivered, choose one of these strategies and apply it to every pregnant woman. Neither of these approaches will prevent 100 percent of cases of GBS, but both will reduce the risk considerably.

Week 35

SUN	DATE
MON	DATE
TUE	DATE
WED	DATE
THUR	DATE
FRI	DATE
SAT	DATE

What Happened This Week?

How I Feel Physically and Emotionally

Here's Looking at You, Kid

THROUGHOUT THIS BOOK, especially when talking about potential complications of pregnancy, I've mentioned *antenatal testing*. Well, now is your chance to learn what this is—this "window on the womb."

What Baby Is Doing

Your baby may start dropping soon. Space is at a premium, and your baby may be starting to feel a bit cramped in his watery room. His fingernails are growing, and he may scratch himself; many a baby is born looking like he shared his space with a cat!

At 35 weeks, your baby is 31 cm (just over a foot) sitting and 44 cm (a foot and a half) all stretched out. He weighs an average of 2,300 gm (he's now a 5-pounder!).

What You Are Doing

This week, when your doctor measures your fundal height (from the top of your pubic bone to the top or your uterus), you may notice it is the same as last week. You may also notice that you are breathing a little easier. If this is the case, it is because your baby is beginning to drop. In first pregnancies, this dropping, technically termed *engagement,* occurs before labor in most cases. If you have already had children, your baby may not drop until you start pushing; in this case, your uterus will continue its centimeter-a-week growth.

You have probably gained 23–28 pounds now, and may be feeling increasingly unwieldy. If the baby's head has dropped, expect frequent trips to the bathroom to start again as the head presses on your bladder. You may also get that late pregnancy waddle.

Special Considerations

If you have experienced any pregnancy complications, or if you have a history of a poor outcome like a stillbirth in the past, your baby will be monitored periodically in the third trimester. This antenatal testing, a.k.a. *antepartum fetal surveillance,* can consist of one or more of several tests. The goal of antenatal testing is to prevent stillbirth and to identify signs of fetal compromise before permanent damage occurs. Indications for antenatal testing are listed in table 35.1.

Most antenatal testing evaluates the baby's heart-rate pattern. Conditions that may adversely affect a developing baby can lead to subtle—and sometimes not so subtle—changes in the normal pattern. Chronic insults (things that happen day in and day out), such as occur with diabetes and high blood pressure or with growth-restricted babies, produce progressive changes in the placenta, including decreased blood flow and delivery of oxygen and nutrients over time, which can be picked up by monitoring techniques. Sudden, catastrophic events like placental abruption or a *cord accident* usually cannot be predicted by antenatal testing.

The first and easiest method of antenatal testing is the *kick count.* Just like it sounds, this involves counting how many times your baby kicks you in a predetermined amount of time. A decrease in movement often precedes a stillbirth by several days, allowing time for additional evaluation and intervention. One way to do a kick count is to lie on your side and count how long it takes the baby to move 10 times (kicks, punches, rolls, wriggles). Do this once a day, preferably after a meal or snack. If it takes more than 2 hours to feel 10 movements, call your doctor. A study out of Denmark showed that this approach significantly reduced the incidence of stillbirth in the group of women doing the kick counts.

The most common means of antenatal testing is the non-stress test (NST). This involves monitoring the baby's heartbeat via a special transducer placed on your belly; usually, a second transducer is used to measure any contractions as well. The technology is the same as the Doppler your doctor uses to listen to your baby's heartbeat, but the information is captured on a strip of paper moving through the monitor. The baby's heartbeat is the top line on the strip, and usually appears squiggly. You may hear your doctor or a nurse say, "The strip looks good," to reflect what the monitoring shows. A completely flat line is ominous. With movement, which you will be asked to indicate by pressing a button, your baby's heart rate should increase, and the strip would be called "reactive." Figure 35.1 shows a reactive NST. If the baby's heart rate does not increase with movement, or if movement cannot be elicited by stimulation (either giving you juice to drink or by acoustic stimulation—placing a vibrating device or artificial larynx over the baby), then the test is deemed "non-reactive," as illustrated in figure 35.2. A non-reactive NST demands additional testing.

If the NST is non-reactive, or in lieu of an NST, a *contraction stress test* (CST) or a *biophysical profile* can give additional information on how your baby is doing. A contraction stress test is pretty much exactly what it sounds like—you are made to contract, and your baby's reaction to the stress of these contractions is monitored exactly as in an NST. Contractions can be elicited by nipple stimulation or by an IV infusion of low-dose *Pitocin*. Because contrac-

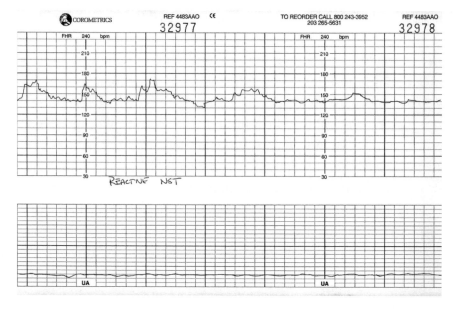

FIGURE 35.1   Reactive NST

Look at how "squiggly" the heart rate is and how it goes up where Mom has indicated she felt the baby move.

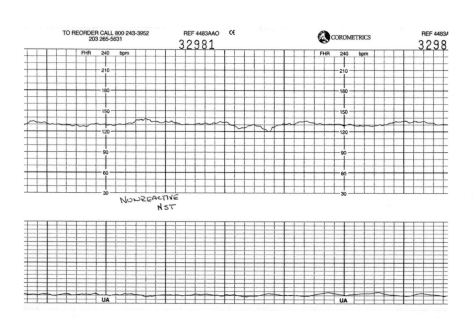

FIGURE 35.2   Nonreactive NST

Notice how flat this strip is compared with the one in figure 35.1.

tions transiently diminish the delivery of oxygen, an already compromised baby will not be able to tolerate any additional decrease in oxygen, and his heart rate will reflect this. Drops in heart rate, called *decelerations*, will occur. *Late decelerations* reflect poor placental function and inadequate oxygenation; they are very worrisome, and if they are repetitive, usually require delivery. Because a CST mimics labor, repetitive late decelerations on a CST (or in labor at any point) usually necessitate a cesarean section. Another type of deceleration that may be seen on the CST is a *variable deceleration*. Variables, to use the common lingo, represent compression of the umbilical cord during a contraction. This can be from the cord being wrapped around the baby's neck (*nuchal cord*), compressed between a body part and the uterine wall if amniotic fluid volume is low, or just from your baby squeezing that funny rope he sees hanging by his face. Mild, intermittent variables are not worrisome, but more consistent or deeper variables demand an assessment of the amniotic fluid volume by ultrasound. Figure 35.3 illustrates the three types of decelerations.

A biophysical profile combines an NST with an ultrasound. The ultrasound is not done to measure how big the baby is or to locate the placenta or check the baby's position, but rather to look at certain things your baby should be doing. Two points are scored for each of the following (partial credit is not given): normal amniotic fluid volume; presence of breathing movements for at least 30 seconds; adequate muscle tone, inferred by seeing either extension and flexion of a limb or opening and closing a hand; and at least 3 discrete movements of the body or limbs in 30 minutes of observation. An additional 2 points is given for a reactive NST. A score of 8 or 10 is normal and indicates there is almost no chance of a stillbirth in the next week. A score of 6 means very close monitoring is necessary, and a score of 4 or less is abnormal, usually leading to a decision to deliver the baby before any further deterioration can occur.

The final form of antenatal testing is *umbilical artery doppler velicometry*, usually called a *doppler flow study*. This test uses a

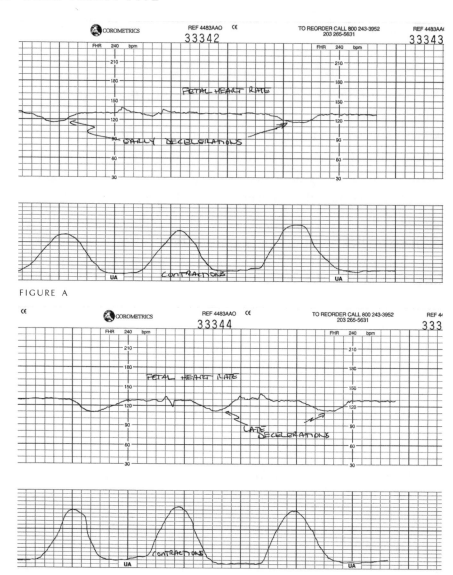

FIGURE A

FIGURE B

FIGURE 35.3 Decelerations

Figure A illustrates an early deceleration, usually associated with head compression during pushing. Notice how it starts when the contraction does and ends as soon as the contraction is over. Figure B is a late deceleration; it is not back to baseline until after the contraction is over; this represents compromised blood flow to the baby. Figure C is a variable deceleration, with a characteristic "V" shape. These usually reflect compression of the umbilical cord.

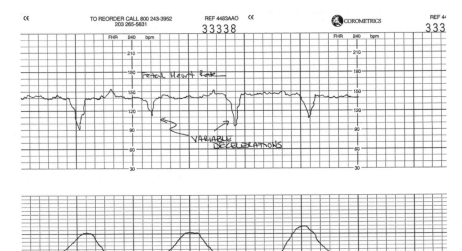

FIGURE C

special type of ultrasound to look at blood flow in your baby's umbilical cord. In babies with IUGR, flow is not normal. If blood flow is absent or in the wrong direction, this is associated with a higher risk of stillbirth, and usually is an indication for delivery. Doppler flow studies are not done as often as the other tests, and there is argument among the experts as to the utility of this test; most agree it should be reserved for babies with IUGR.

When testing is started and how often it is done depends on the reason the test is being done in the first place. In most cases, antenatal testing is begun around 32 weeks, although in cases of poorly controlled insulin dependent diabetes, IUGR, or severe hypertension, testing may be initiated around 28 weeks. Most of the time the test—probably an NST—is repeated weekly. Again, in poorly controlled diabetes, pre-eclampsia, or IUGR, the testing may be done twice a week. If your baby continues to look good on the testing, delivery can be delayed until you are closer to your due date or the cervix becomes more favorable of a vaginal delivery. If at any point your baby "flunks" a CST or biophysical profile, delivery will be accomplished; whether that occurs by inducing labor or perform-

TABLE 35.1

Indications for Antenatal Testing

Maternal Conditions

Antiphospholipid syndrome

Chronic high blood pressure

Chronic kidney disease (usually accompanied by hypertension)

Insulin dependent diabetes

Sickle cell disease and other hemoglobinopathies

Stage III or IV heart disease

Fetal/Pregnancy Related Conditions

Decreased fetal movement

Isoimmunization due to Rh or other factors

Oligohydramnios

Polyhydramnios

Postdates (> 42 weeks) pregnancy

Pre-eclampsia

Prior stillbirth

Twins or more, if there is growth discrepancy between the babies

IUGR

ing a cesarean section depends on your individual circumstances and exactly how worrisome the monitoring is.

Antenatal testing is a good way to get a "window on the womb" to see how your baby is tolerating her environment and to predict how she will do in labor. As I mentioned before, it cannot prevent all stillbirths or bad outcomes, because sudden, unpredictable events like a placental abruption or the baby's cord knotting usually do not give any warning signs. Still, in the conditions for which antenatal testing is indicated, it can make a difference in your baby's health.

Frequently Asked Questions

Q This week, when the doctor measured me, I still measured 34 cm. Until now, I've been measuring exactly how many weeks I am. Does this mean the baby isn't growing any more? By the way, I'm also having to go to the bathroom more.

A *If you've also noticed it's a bit easier to breathe, this apparent lack of change in your fundal height may just mean the baby is starting to drop. The rule about the fundal height (in centimeters) equaling the weeks of pregnancy holds only from 20 to 34 weeks. After the thirty-fourth week, the height may not increase as much as the baby drops lower in the pelvis. It is the pressure of the baby's head on your pelvis that is causing more trips to the bathroom.*

If your doctor is concerned that the lack of growth in your uterus is due to the baby not growing well, she will order an ultrasound. But, given the timing and the increased pressure you're feeling, this is probably just the baby dropping.

Q My baby has IUGR, and I've been having twice a week NSTs for several weeks now. They've looked great until this last one, so the doctor did a biophysical profile. She said everything was good except the amniotic fluid was low, and gave the baby a score of 6 out of a possible 10. I have to have another biophysical profile tomorrow. What's going to happen if the baby gets a 6 again?

A *If a baby scores 6 on a biophysical profile and the baby is not yet term, the test is repeated in 24 hours. Sometimes, a contraction stress test may be done, either in addition to or in place of the repeat biophysical profile. If your baby, at 35 weeks, scores 6 or less again today, your doctor will probably recommend delivery. Most of the time, a vaginal delivery can be attempted, but if your baby does not handle the contractions well, a cesarean will be done. Babies with IUGR are stressed in the womb, and while in general stress is not a good thing, one advantage of exposure to a stressful environment is that your baby's lungs mature faster. A baby with IUGR usually does not have the same need for supplemental oxygen as another baby who does not have IUGR born at the same gestational age.*

Q I have to have a contraction stress test because of equivocal findings on an NST and the fact that I have high blood pressure. The nurse in my doctor's office said I'll do a nipple stimulation. What exactly does that mean?

A *Stimulating your nipples mimics a baby nursing and causes oxytocin to be released from your brain. Oxytocin is important in milk let-down and also causes the uterus to contract. Nipple stimulation has been found to produce an adequate contraction pattern in less time than using IV Pitocin.*

First, you are put on the monitor. Belts or a length of stretchy material (think tube top) are placed on your belly to hold the transducers (think hockey puck) that will record your baby's heartbeat and the contractions (this is the same as an NST). You will be monitored for 10–20 minutes to get your baby's baseline heartbeat and also to see if you are having spontaneous contractions. If you are not contracting, you will begin the nipple stimulation. You will be asked to rub your nipple through your clothing or with a washcloth for 2 minutes, or until a contraction starts. If after that, you don't start having contractions at a frequency of 3 in 10 minutes, you rest for 5 minutes and start rubbing your nipple again. If this does not start an adequate contraction pattern after a few tries, you will have an IV started and be given dilute Pitocin instead.

Contraction stress tests are generally not done in women with preterm labor or at high risk for preterm labor; preterm rupture of the membranes; prior myomectomy or classical (vertical uterine incision) cesarean section (due to risk of the uterine scar rupturing, these women are not allowed to labor but rather have scheduled cesarean sections); placenta previa (to avoid contractions that may cause catastrophic bleeding).

Week 36

SUN _____ DATE

MON _____ DATE

TUE _____ DATE

WED _____ DATE

THUR _____ DATE

FRI _____ DATE

SAT _____ DATE

_____

What Happened This Week?

_____

_____

_____

_____

How I Feel Physically and Emotionally

_____

_____

_____

_____

To Breast or Not to Breast, That Is the Question

WHETHER 'TIS NOBLER to breastfeed is a matter of great debate today among women in this country. Breast milk is unequivocally beneficial for babies, but formula is not harmful. Breast or bottle is a personal choice, and one is not "nobler" than the other.

What Baby Is Doing

Your little one has plump cheeks—and a roly-poly body to go along with them. The cheeks are so well developed because your baby has been sucking her thumb, fist, toes, and anything else she can get in her mouth in preparation for nursing; once she's out, she's going to have to work a bit to get her food.

Your baby weighs, on average, 2,500 gm (5 lbs. 8 oz.) and is 45 cm (18 in) tall.

What You Are Doing

You are in the home stretch now—only 4 short weeks until your due date, although it probably feels like forever! You are probably

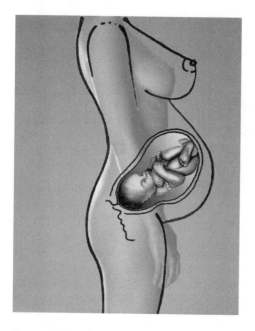

You are 36 weeks—in the home stretch. Your uterus may not grow much more as the baby settles into your pelvis in preparation for delivery day.

anxious to see your little passenger. Your baby's movements may feel different now, as his space is increasingly cramped. Instead of somersaults, you may feel more rolls and stretches, or the jab of a knee or elbow.

Your feet and ankles may be swollen from the pressure of your rather large uterus. Some degree of swelling is normal, and is usually alleviated by putting your feet up a couple of times a day, but if you have massive swelling or swelling of your hands and face, or a bad head-ache, be sure to call your doctor. These could be signs of pre-eclampsia.

Special Considerations

The American College of Obstetricians and Gynecologists (ACOG), along with the World Health Organization (WHO) and the American Academy of Pediatrics (AAP), recommends exclusive breastfeeding for the first 6 months of life. AAP goes on to recommend that breastfeeding continue for at least 12 months, and thereafter for as long as both you and your baby desire. This may seem like a Herculean task, but it is doable. I am a very busy doctor. I write weekly columns for several Internet sites. I am the spokesperson for First Response. I breastfed my daughter for 12 months and 2 weeks, until she weaned herself, much to my dismay—she was ready but I wasn't. It is not always easy to pump so that your child can get breast milk from a bottle while you are at work, but it can be done.

From My Journal

"11/14/98. You are 36 4/7 weeks and I am 38 years old today! You looked great on the last ultrasound 2 days ago—good fluid, placenta not too calcified, weight 2,588 gms [5 lbs. 11 oz.]. I stopped the heparin yesterday [I was taking heparin, a blood thinner, by injection twice a day since conception due to antiphospholipid syndrome, which can cause tiny blood clots in the placenta, increasing the risk of miscarriage and stillbirth]. I am so looking forward to your birth. I can't wait to hold you. Your dad is anxious—he's worried about something going wrong. I was the anxious one earlier, but now he is the worrywart! He wants me to have an NST every day! On my NST today I was having contractions—couldn't even feel them, and only palpated mild when I noticed them on the strip. I hope they are doing something. . . . We're going to Evan's [a favorite local restaurant] for my birthday dinner, so you'll get a nice meal."

The benefits to your baby from breastfeeding are numerous, and have been substantiated through research throughout the world. Human milk provides nutrients needed by human babies. Breast milk changes as your baby grows and is adapted to meet the needs of your baby at each stage of life. Iron is present in lower amounts in breast milk than in formula, but the iron in breast milk is so readily absorbed that only premature newborns and babies whose mothers are anemic need supplementary iron. Colostrum, the milk produced immediately after birth, is high in immunoglobulins. This offers protection against infections. Breastfed babies are less likely to have diarrhea, respiratory infections, and earaches.

Breastfed babies are less likely to develop diabetes, allergies, obesity, lymphoma, Crohn's disease, and ulcerative colitis. Breastfed babies are less likely to suffer SIDS (sudden infant death syndrome, a.k.a. crib death). If that isn't an argument to breastfeed, I don't know what is!

There are benefits to you, too. Oxytocin released as your baby nurses causes your uterus to contract, decreasing blood loss. I don't know whether it was the breastfeeding or just plain good luck, but I only bled—and lightly at that—for 2 weeks after I gave birth. Oxytocin also seems to lead to a sensation of relaxation and well-being; believe me, you first-time moms-to-be, you'll need all the help you can get in this department! Breastfeeding lowers the chance of you developing breast cancer, although for us over-35-year-olds, that effect is not as pronounced as it is in younger women. Breast milk is free. Even if you work, and have to buy bottles to give your baby expressed breast milk, and even if you buy the fanciest double electric breast pump, it is still less expensive than formula. And, here is the reason you may find the most motivating to breastfeed: Breastfeeding helps you lose your pregnancy weight faster.

Many women are leery of breastfeeding, feeling it will tie them down too much. Yes, you will either have to plan solo excursions around baby's feeding times or pump and leave a bottle of breast milk. But, when you do take your baby with you, your breasts are always there, too. No bottles to clean, no formula to mix and heat. It is so easy to give your baby exactly the right amount of milk at exactly the right temperature, no matter where you are when your baby is hungry. I nursed my daughter in Nordstrom's ladies' lounge (my favorite spot!), in my car, on airplanes, in restaurants, in hospital meetings (my male colleagues were not fazed by me nursing at the conference table, but they had a fit when I changed Hunter's diaper in the corner of the room!), and smack dab in the middle of Costco (those display lounge chairs come in handy!).

Almost every woman can nurse. The size of your breasts is not correlated with how much milk you produce. Women with flat or inverted nipples can usually breastfeed as well. Sometimes, breast shields are used during the last several weeks of pregnancy to help draw out inverted nipples. Using a breast pump for a few minutes prior to nursing can also help draw nipples out so your baby can latch on properly. If you must return to work shortly after your baby is born, or if your baby is premature and cannot latch on and nurse, you can pump and give your baby all the benefits of breast milk in a bottle.

If you have HIV, you should not breastfeed. If you have hepatitis, once your baby gets the immune globulin shot and vaccine, you can breastfeed. Many medications are okay to use while breastfeeding, but always let your doctor know you are nursing so the safest choice can be prescribed.

I am going to tell it to you straight: Sometimes nursing hurts like hell. All the breastfeeding books I read (and I read several) talked about discomfort if the baby didn't latch on properly, or if your nipples got cracked (usually from improper latch-on). Well, ladies, discomfort is an understatement. If your baby is not latched on properly, or if you have cracked nipples, it hurts. *Pain.* I had cracked nipples for about 3 weeks before I gave my pride the boot and called a lactation consultant for help (remember, I'm the doctor; I'm supposed to be giving, not getting, help!). Hunter cried because she was hungry, and then I cried when she latched on. My poor husband just rubbed my back and brought me the Lansinoh. Purified lanolin like Lansinoh should be in every nursing mom's medicine cabinet. So should a heating pad for blocked milk ducts. I had that, too. Holding your baby in different positions so she can empty all the ducts, massaging your breasts while the baby is nursing, using hot compresses or a heating pad, or letting hot water beat on the clogged area can help keep a blocked duct from progressing to the more serious *mastitis*. Mastitis is a breast infection, heralded by a very sore, red, warm area on your breasts, and accompanied by fever and just generally not feeling well. Blocked ducts do not require antibiotics; mastitis does. Given that, nursing my daughter for a year was one of the most rewarding and fulfilling experiences of my life, and one that I miss now that she is a very independent toddler.

So, if women have been breastfeeding since the dawn of time (there was no formula in those caves, after all), then it must come naturally and easily. Wrong. Years ago, women had their mothers and their grandmothers and the village medicine woman to help them with their newborns. Today, we go home 12 hours after giving birth and expect to handle it all. Heck, you are a mature, motivated, successful woman; surely you can figure it out! What you need to figure out is who to ask for assistance. I am a great believer in both lactation consultants and the La Leche League. Lactation consultants are trained to assist you with all your nursing concerns, from proper latching on, to breast pump selection and rental, to ways to up your milk supply. La Leche League leaders and the women who attend the meeting are also wonderful sources of information, but more important, they form an invaluable support network. I attended many La Leche League meetings and enjoyed the company of other nursing moms. I got tips not only on successful breastfeeding but on all sorts of other parenting concerns. The La Leche League's toll-free number is 1-800-LA LECHE, and their Web site is *www.lalecheleague.org*. The La Leche League book, *The Womanly Art of Breastfeeding*, Karen Huggins's *The Nursing Mother's Companion*, and *The Complete Book of Breastfeeding* by Eiger and Olds were kept close at hand, on a table next to the glider where I nursed Hunter, along with Dr. Spock, Dr. Brazelton, a water bottle, a cordless phone, and that Lansinoh!

In 1998, 64.3 percent of mothers left the hospital breastfeeding their babies. Only 28.6 percent were still breastfeeding at the 6-month mark, and this was the highest rate in the 30 years such data has been gathered.

Obviously, if you are not going to breastfeed, you will be using formula. Choosing to give your baby formula rather than the breast is not evil, although some advocates of breastfeeding may make you feel that way. Formula provides adequate nutrition, although it does not have the immune-enhancing properties of breast milk. You can bond with your baby just as well as a nursing mom if you avoid bad habits like propping the bottle and instead snuggle close with your little one. Using formula allows you more freedom and gives dads, grandmas, and grandpas the opportunity to feed the baby as well (as does bottle feeding pumped breast milk).

If you are on the fence about breastfeeding, I would encourage you to give it a try. See a lactation consultant or attend a La Leche League meeting before you deliver. Ask the nurses at the hospital to help you once you give birth; many hospitals have lactation consultants on staff to provide assistance. If you cannot or do not want to breastfeed, be sure to wear a snugly fitting bra to avoid engorgement, and avoid any stimulation of your nipples. Tylenol and a cool compress (cold cabbage leaves inside your bra work well) will help you get over the worst of it on the third or fourth day after you deliver your baby. Whatever you do, if you choose not to breastfeed, don't squeeze your breasts! You may think if you relieve some of the pressure, it will feel so much better, but your breasts are going to think a baby is eating and they'll just keep making milk. And you'll just keep being miserable.

Frequently Asked Questions

Q I have breast implants. Will I be able to nurse? And will the silicone cause any harm (I'm 40 and got my implants 20 years ago)?

A *Most women with breast implants can successfully nurse their babies. Most of the time, the incision is in the armpit or under the breast, and it does not interfere with major nerves or milk ducts. Even if an incision is made around the areola, as long as all milk ducts are not severed, breastfeeding can occur. There is no good evidence that silicone leaks into breast milk from intact implants or causes any harm to babies.*

Q I had a breast reduction several years ago. I nursed my first two children without any problem, but I'm wondering if I'll be able to breastfeed this one.

A *Many of the techniques used in breast reduction surgery today will allow you to attempt breastfeeding. If, however, all the nerves and ducts going to the areola-nipple complex were severed, you will not be able to nurse. If you attempt breastfeeding, your baby will need to be closely monitored to make sure he is getting adequate amounts of milk. Sometimes you will be able to supply a little, but not enough to meet all of your baby's needs; you can nurse first, and then give a supplemental bottle of formula.*

Q I plan to try breastfeeding, but I'm worried I won't make enough milk. How will I know if my baby is getting enough?

A *This is a concern of many women, because breasts are not transparent and they don't have ounce markings on them! There are several ways to tell whether your baby is getting enough breast milk. In the first few weeks of life, your baby should nurse 8–10 times a day, for 10–20 minutes on each breast. She should sleep 1–3 hours between feedings if her needs are being met. She should have more than six wet diapers a day, and the urine should be pale yellow if she is getting enough fluid. Her bowel movements should be regular— although with breastfeeding, regular could mean once a day or, as was the case with my daughter, after every feeding! Her skin should be smooth and plump, and she should be alert and bright-eyed.*

If you notice your baby is not wetting many diapers, seems listless, or cries all the time, even after nursing, see your pediatrician. You may need to bring her in to be weighed several times to ensure she is getting enough milk and growing properly. This was a big concern of mine. Hunter only weighed 5 lbs. 13 oz. at birth, had dropped down to 5 lb. 6 oz., and I was sure I wasn't going to produce enough milk. By 17 days of life, she was up to 7 lbs. 1 oz., had grown 1½ inches, and I stopped worrying about inadequate production!

Q I really want to breastfeed but I have to go back to work when my baby will be 6 weeks old. I can pump during my breaks, but my boss has said I can only take two 20-minute breaks a day, plus lunch. Can I pump in that amount of time? And will this be enough to leave the amount of milk my baby needs?

A *If you are serious about wanting to give your baby breast milk, you can do it. First, either buy or rent a hospital-grade double electric breast pump. By pumping both your breasts simultaneously, you will be able to extract the most milk in the least amount of time. I bought the Medela Pump In Style, and I could empty both breasts in about 12 minutes (my office scheduled 15-minute "pump breaks" into my day, one in mid-morning and one mid-afternoon; I used a special bra, hooked the pump up, and made phone calls—I now truly know how cows feel at milking time!). If you cannot get home—or have your baby brought to you—at lunch, pump again then. Store the milk in a refrigerator or in a small cooler with ice packs. Because of its anti-bacterial properties, breast milk will keep at room temperature for up to 10 hours. It can be refrigerated for 8 days and frozen for up to 6 months without losing any nutritional value. What you pump today can be given to baby the next workday. I did this for a year, while working in the office 3–4 days a week and doing surgery 1 day a week. After a while, it becomes routine, although hearing "Take your time cleaning the room. Dr. Shanahan's going to get milked" over the OR intercom was something I never got used to!*

Week 37

SUN _____ DATE _____

MON _____ DATE _____

TUE _____ DATE _____

WED _____ DATE _____

THUR _____ DATE _____

FRI _____ DATE _____

SAT _____ DATE _____

What Happened This Week?

_____

_____

_____

_____

How I Feel Physically and Emotionally

_____

_____

_____

_____

The Home Stretch

Your DUE DATE is so close you can smell it. As of this week your baby is considered full-term! If you were on bed rest or medication for preterm labor, you can stop the meds and get out of bed. If you had a cerclage for an incompetent cervix, it will be removed this week. If you haven't gotten a car seat yet, you better get hopping. Baby's birth is just around the corner!

What Baby Is Doing

He may not have a calendar on the wall of his home, and he may not be counting down the days, but your baby is getting ready for birth, too. He is putting on about an ounce per day now, fat stores to supply his needs until your milk comes in. In his nervous system, *myelin,* a protective sheath, is forming around nerves; this will continue throughout the first year of life, allowing more efficient and coordinated movements as development progresses. Surfactant production in the lungs is in full swing, in preparation for breathing air in a matter of days or a few short weeks.

Your 37-week-old baby should weigh 2,700 gm (5 lbs. 14 oz.). Sitting, he is 33 cm (13 in), and from head to toe he is almost 19 inches long.

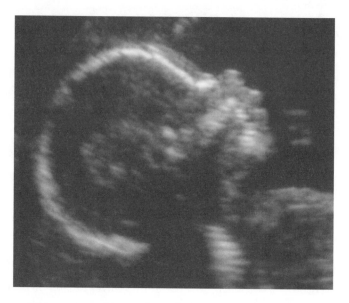

"He's got your chin—and grandpa's nose. A profile in utero."

What You Are Doing

You will be seeing your doctor every week now until your baby is born. Because pre-eclampsia is much more likely to rear its ugly head in the last few weeks of pregnancy, your blood pressure will need to be monitored. By feeling your belly, your doctor can tell if the baby is head first or breech, and may be able to give you a "guesstimate" of your baby's weight. This estimate is give or take a pound and is not exact. You may also have a pelvic exam every week to see if your cervix is beginning to dilate or efface. Don't get too excited if your doctor tells you that you are a centimeter or 2 dilated; you can walk around for weeks that way. I wish the onset of labor could be predicted based on how dilated you are (I'd win all the baby pools that way!), but the baby will come when she is ready—not when you are.

Special Considerations

You are ready for your baby's arrival. You've taken the classes, the nursery is freshly painted and decorated (and thoroughly aired out!), the crib is up. You are all set. You think you are all set. You hope you are all set. You've never done this before (or you did it 20 years ago), so you panic, wondering if everything is ready for your baby. Stop, take a deep breath, and relax. While a perfectly organized and beautifully decorated nursery is a wonderful thing, your baby won't care if the bedding matches the wallpaper or not. All you really need are diapers (lots of diapers), the items from the following list, and a good sense of humor. Baby can sleep in a drawer taken out of the dresser and placed on the floor if need be. I think my mom said she put me in a dresser drawer when she first brought me home from the hospital, and I turned out okay!

There are advantages to doing as much as possible before your baby is out in the world. First and foremost, it is a lot easier to accomplish a task if you do not have to haul a newborn, a diaper bag, and three changes of clothing to the store to buy diapers. Second, you are much more likely to put the crib together correctly if you haven't been up every 2 hours feeding, burping, and changing poopy diapers. Third, who wants to wash new baby clothes when you can stare at your baby's beautiful face instead?

When making purchases for your baby, your number one priority should be safety. If you want to go for designer or budget next, feel free, but make sure everything you purchase for your baby is the best in terms of safety. I took Consumer Reports' Guide to Baby Products to every store. I researched cribs and mattresses and high chairs and car seats and strollers before I whipped out the Discover card. Buying secondhand or using hand-me-downs is perfectly fine for most items, but do invest in a new, highly rated car seat. If you get a used crib, bring a measuring tape to make sure the slats are no more than 2⅜ inches apart and the mattress fits snugly, with no gaps into which the baby could fall.

You could buy baby things for days on end, and still see some adorable little outfit or toy or gadget. Here's what you need, bare bones, no frills:

CLOTHING

- 3–7 undershirts. Personally, I like the snap-crotch body suits, but then, my daughter was born in Tahoe in December.
- 3–7 nightgowns with drawstring, elastic, or snap bottoms. Guess what? You can keep the baby in this all day. The open bottom makes diaper changes easy.
- 3–7 pairs of socks or booties, for keeping tiny tootsies toasty.
- 1–3 blanket sleepers. For a winter baby, these are much safer than using a blanket over baby. A summer baby can get by with just the nightgown or stretchie.
- 3–5 stretchies with feet for a fall or winter baby, or 3–6 rompers for a spring or summer baby.
- 1–3 hats. A hat with a big brim is a must for summer babies who are going to be outside; winter babies need a snug knit or fleece hat to keep head and ears warm.
- 1–3 sweaters. Lightweight for a summer baby, heavier for a winter one. If you live in a cold climate, a bunting is great to keep your baby warm on winter walks.

LINENS

- 3–6 receiving blankets.
- 3–4 fitted crib sheets for crib and bassinet.
- 2–4 waterproof pads for protecting crib, bassinet, and whatever else you don't want to get wet from urine, stool, spit up, and all the other fluids that leak from newborns.
- 1–2 blankets for the stroller or walking out to the mailbox.
- 2–3 washcloths and hooded towels.
- 12 cloth diapers. Even if you are going to use disposable diapers, these make great burp cloths. I left the house one day and

went to the office with one on my shoulder. What a fashion statement!

- 3–6 bibs. Even newborns drool a lot.

TOILETRIES

- 1 bottle of baby bath liquid and 1 of baby shampoo. I bought the great big bottle of Johnson & Johnson shampoo at Costco, and I'm still using it 21 months later!
- Baby tub. I swear by the Century Cuddle Tub. It has a hammock the baby rests in to help decrease your fears of trying to hold on to a wet, slippery baby.
- 1 tube diaper rash ointment. It also comes in handy if you get irritated or chafed from wearing pads after delivery—in fact, I used the Desitin before Hunter did!
- 1 small jar petroleum jelly, for lubricating a rectal thermometer.
- 1 rectal thermometer. For newborns, they are the most accurate.
- Diaper wipes or cotton balls and warm water. I found cotton balls and warm water much less irritating to my daughter's delicate bottom—I kept a Pyrex bowl with water on a coffee mug warmer on her changing table. I bought cotton balls by the gross at—where else!—Costco.
- Diapers. 2–5 dozen cloth or several dozen disposable. If you use cloth diapers, line up a diaper service before you deliver, and buy 3–4 diaper wraps as well.
- 1 baby nail clipper. I do surgery for a living, but I was scared to death to clip my daughter's nails!
- Baby brush and comb. If you are lucky enough to have a child with hair. Otherwise, you can pretend and just gently brush that bald scalp.
- 1 bottle baby acetominophen (Tylenol).
- Nasal aspirator, for a stuffy nose.
- Cool mist vaporizer or humidifier, especially in a dry climate or

in a house heated with forced-air heat. This helps keep your baby's nasal passages from drying out.

FEEDING

- 1 pair of breasts and Lansinoh for you.
- 8–12 4-ounce bottles, with nipples if you are bottlefeeding (you'll need the 8-ounce bottles later). 4–6 bottles if you are nursing but planning to pump.
- Bottle brushes.

FURNITURE

- 1 bassinet or cradle. Even if you are planning on keeping your baby in bed with you, a bassinet is a nice, portable place to put baby for a nap.
- 1 crib with mattress and bumpers. The crib looked so lovely in Hunter's room, but for the first 6 months of her life, it was a repository for stuffed animals while she slept in her $50 bassinet!
- Changing table. I used—and still do—the top of her dresser.
- Dresser or chest of drawers. Can double as a changing table if it's about waist high.
- Rocking chair or glider. A great place to nurse the baby or rock to soothe her—and you.
- Diaper pail. I like the Diaper Genie for keeping odors down.

LEAVING THE HOUSE

- Car seat. Go for the safest one here. In *Consumer Reports,* the safest one listed is not the most expensive, either. Baby needs to face the rear until she is 1 year old and more than 20 pounds. I liked an infant carrier/car seat that fit into a base that stayed in the car. We ordered an extra base for my husband's truck, to make for smooth transfers if I had to hand her over to him while I went to do a delivery.

- Stroller or carriage. My car seat also fit onto the stroller, which is great for shopping—you don't have to wake baby up, just take the carrier/car seat out of the car and pop it on the stroller. They often fit on grocery carts, too.
- Diaper bag. Look for multiple compartments to help keep all the supplies organized. I like a backpack model because it keeps my hands free.
- Front pack or sling. We couldn't have survived without these. I wore Hunter in the sling all day, and Jeff took her cross-country skiing in the front pack when she was 10 days old.

Isn't it amazing how much stuff you'll need for such a little person? And this list doesn't even cover mobiles, stuffed animals, rattles, and those precious little outfits!

In addition to making sure everything is in order for your baby, you will have to make sure you have a few things to bring to the hospital. Before you pack your bag, take some time to make sure all bills are up to date, arrangements have been made for other children (and pets) when you are at the hospital, there is film in the camera, and you have compiled a list of telephone numbers and e-mail addresses of the people you want to notify. Following is a list of things to bring with you, without having to rent a U-Haul.

HOSPITAL PACKING LIST

- Address book and calling card
- Baby book to get footprints
- Birth plan (if you wrote one)
- Body pillow, or a couple of your favorite pillows
- Books or magazines (if your labor is induced, you are going to want something to do)
- Bunting or heavy blanket (if it is cold), to cover baby on the trip home
- Camera (still and/or video)

- Candles or aromatherapy (if your hospital will allow it)
- Car seat (make sure you've tested it in your car before it's time to take baby home!)
- CD or cassette player with music you like
- Hard candy and popsicles
- Hat for baby
- Insurance card and forms
- Loose, comfortable clothing to wear going home (leave the jeans in the closet, sorry)
- Baby outfit for homecoming picture
- Picture or other focal point you have chosen
- Receiving blanket
- Robe, pajamas/nightgown, and underwear
- Snacks for dad
- Tennis ball or rolling pin (great for back during labor)
- Toiletries (brush, comb, toothbrush and paste, glasses or contact lenses, shampoo)

Frequently Asked Questions

Q When my doctor measured me today, she also felt for the baby's position. She thought—and later an ultrasound confirmed—the baby was breech. She said she would try to turn the baby later this week. How is that done?

A *Your doctor is referring to an* external cephalic version. *This is done in the hospital, as there is a small risk of causing fetal distress and needing to perform an emergency cesarean section. Often an IV is started, just in case. First, you will have an NST to make sure the baby is not stressed already. An ultrasound will be done to confirm your baby's position and to check for the location of the placenta. It is best if the placenta is on the back wall of the uterus; this location diminishes the risk of shearing off the placenta while maneuvering the baby, and also makes it easier to get a grip on the baby. The doctor will also* look for an adequate amount of amniotic fluid, as too little fluid makes it difficult to turn the baby. You may be given a shot of terbutaline to prevent contractions during the version. No pain medication will be given, because if the doctor is pushing and prodding so hard as to cause significant pain, the risk of injuring you and the baby is too high and the attempt is stopped.

Your doctor will use a small amount of lubricant on your belly to reduce friction, but not enough so that she can't get a grip on the baby. She will gently grasp your baby's buttocks with one hand and the head with the other and try to roll the baby forward, guiding the head into your pelvis. Versions are successful about 65 percent of the time. If the baby will not flip after several attempts, either a cesarean section will be planned or your doctor will discuss an attempt at vaginal breech delivery (this latter option is usually only given in the United States if you have already had children. The vast majority of first-time moms with a breech baby will have cesarean sections).

Q This is my second child. I had to be induced 2 weeks after my due date last time, but I'm already 2 cm dilated. I haven't even noticed any contractions. Does this mean I'll deliver soon?

A Sorry, but being 2 or even 4 centimeters dilated does not predict when you will go into labor and deliver. I've had patients walk around 4 centimeters dilated for more than 3 weeks. Losing the mucus plug, despite what you may have heard from your mother, does not mean labor is going to start soon, either.

If you are dilated your doctor may ask if you want your membranes stripped. This is not the same as rupturing the membranes, but rather involves the doctor running her finger around the inner edge of your dilated cervix, separating the membranes from the underlying uterine wall. The theory is that this may stimulate release of prostaglandins that may help initiate labor. Stripping of the membranes does not mean labor will start soon, but it does lower the chance you'll be late.

Week 38

SUN _____ DATE _____

MON _____ DATE _____

TUE _____ DATE _____

WED _____ DATE _____

THUR _____ DATE _____

FRI _____ DATE _____

SAT _____ DATE _____

What Happened This Week?

_____

_____

_____

How I Feel Physically and Emotionally

_____

_____

_____

_____

Pain Control

You have taken childbirth classes and you want an unmedicated birth, but you are afraid you won't be able to do it when push comes to shove. You know you are a wimp, and you want an epidural as soon as you are admitted. At every stage of labor, there are options for dealing with the pain; no option is good or bad, but you need to know what they are in order to make an intelligent, informed decision about which to choose.

What Baby Is Doing

Your baby has lost the lanugo hair that covered her body only a few weeks ago. Vernix is still present, but not in such abundant amounts. Her toenails reach the ends of her toes. She is ready and waiting to be born.

If your baby were born now (and she well could be), she'd have a crown–rump length of 34 cm (almost 14 in) and be about 48 cm (19 in) tall. Average weight at 38 weeks is 2,900 gm (6 lbs. 5 oz.), but there is considerable variation. Babies' birthweights are often the average of their parents' weights at birth.

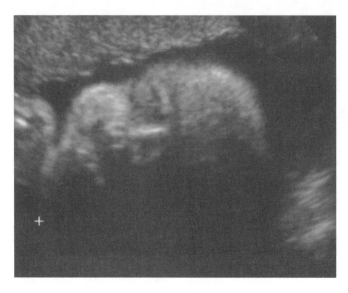

"A face to launch a thousand smiles. . ."

What You Are Doing

Besides pacing the floor waiting for your baby to be born, you may be experiencing an increasing number of Braxton Hicks contractions. You may start frantically timing them, hoping it's the real thing, only to find yourself sleeping with a pad of paper on your chest (you haven't had a lap for a long time!). You are probably having to get up in the night to empty your bladder; pressure from your baby's head means you can't hold much urine. You may also become incontinent if you laugh, cough, sneeze, or are just too far from a bathroom when the urge strikes. If you aren't sure whether you lost urine or broke your water bag, be sure to call your doctor; better to be sent home with Depends than to ignore ruptured membranes and risk a serious infection.

Special Considerations

Some women can get through labor without breaking a sweat or smearing their make-up. Others are screaming for drugs at 1 centimeter. The vast majority are somewhere in between. I encourage open-mindedness about pain relief in labor. If this is your first baby, you don't know what your tolerance to contractions will be. I have delivered thousands of babies, so I've certainly had a lot of experience with what labor and delivery are like. I have had two major abdominal surgeries and a bowel obstruction as a child, thanks to a trampoline accident. I thought labor would be a piece of cake compared to the bowel obstruction. Wrong. I do have a high pain threshold, but after being stuck at 5 centimeters for a couple of hours, my attempts at self-hypnosis and breathing could no longer handle the pain of my contractions. Choosing an epidural at that point enabled me to enjoy the next hour and gave me the strength to push my daughter out when the time came. At the same time, I am proud of myself for getting as far as I did without any pain medication, and do not see getting an epidural as a "failure"—how could anything that helped me bring my wonderful daughter into the world be considered failing?

Let's talk about what the options are for pain control in labor, starting from the least interventional to the most. The least invasive method of pain control in labor lies within you—your inner strength. By tapping into this potential, by learning how to accept the sensations you are feeling, you may be able to give birth without any drugs or an epidural. Classes like Bradley and Lamaze may help you find ways to achieve this. Hypnosis is another very effective means of having a relatively pain-free labor. I tried it, but it didn't work for me, probably because I did not dedicate enough time and effort to it in the last couple of months before delivering— it takes more than two sessions in the 2 weeks before your due date to be successful with hypnosis!

Acupuncture or acupressure can also help with contraction pain. If your hospital does not have someone trained in acupuncture on staff (and 99 percent don't) or will not allow an outside acupuncturist to come in (for liability reasons), you could see a licensed acupuncturist before giving birth so that you and your coach can learn some acupressure techniques. In Asia, acupuncture is used for surgical anesthesia, so it is a potent force in pain relief. Along the same lines as acupuncture is use of a TENS (*transcutaneous electrical nerve stimulation*). Small electrodes are placed to stimulate the nerves supplying the uterus and vagina. This stimulation may block transmission of pain sensations—like the Klingons jamming Star Fleet transmissions. You control the intensity of stimulation to suit what you are feeling at that particular time.

Intravenous narcotics are another option, but since they do cross the placenta and can affect the baby, they are best reserved for earlier in labor. If narcotics are given too close to the time your baby is born, the baby can be *depressed,* meaning it has poor muscle tone and does not make good breathing efforts. If this occurs, your baby will be given a shot of Narcan (naloxone) to reverse the effects of the narcotic. Narcotics do not take the pain away completely, but rather "take the edge off." You may be able to drift off between contractions, but you will still feel them. Sometimes, narcotics may make you nauseated; other medication can be given to combat this if it does happen. Common narcotics used in labor are listed in table 38.1.

The final type of labor analgesic is a "regional block," better known as an *epidural* or a *spinal.* There are differences between the two; an epidural is the most commonly used, although spinals are most often used for cesarean sections (and will be discussed in week 39). When a patient has been struggling with her labor and decides on an epidural, I tell her that the anesthesiologist who administers it is going to be her new best friend. An epidural involves the anesthesiologist using a long, skinny needle to guide an even longer, skinnier catheter into the space just outside the *dura,* the membranous covering of the spinal cord. By injecting a local anesthetic (one of many of the "-caines" related to novacaine) and sometimes a narcotic as well, the nerves to the uterus—and everything below—are numbed. You may notice that your legs feel heavy and warm, and you may not be able to move them well, especially if a straight "-caine" is used. You will also notice your contractions are no longer painful, although you may have a sensation of your uterus tightening or may feel some rectal pressure if you are fully dilated and your baby's head is very low. If a mix of narcotic and a bit of local anesthetic is used, sometimes called an *epidural light,* you may be able to control your legs and feel your contractions, but they won't be perceived as painful. A *walking epidural* is actually a combination of narcotics injected directly into the spinal fluid (providing about 2 hours of pain relief without interfering with your ability to move); an epidural catheter is left in place in case further analgesia is needed once the spinal begins to wear off.

There is a lot of debate about the best time in labor to give an epidural. Given too soon, it can interfere with the normal progress of labor. Wait too long and the baby may be out before you get it (in which case you probably didn't need it anyway!). Ideally, I like to wait until you are at least 4 centimeters dilated; given at this point or beyond, the epidural is less likely to slow down labor or interfere with the descent of the baby's head. As far as I'm concerned, you can get an epidural up until you feel the urge to push—at that point, if you are fully dilated and the baby's head is so low you feel rectal pressure, that kid will be out before an epidural could take effect.

Because of the anatomy of the epidural space, you may not get 100 percent even relief—the epidural may be "patchy." There may be one small area where you still feel pain. Sometimes by adjusting the catheter, this can be fixed. Another potential problem with an epidural is that you may not notice the sensations of a full bladder, and may not be able to empty your bladder even if you did. If this occurs, a catheter will be placed to drain urine. Because not every woman has urinary retention, I don't think every woman with an epidural needs a catheter as a matter of routine—I believe in the wait-and-see-what-happens approach. I for one had a very dense epidural, but had no problem urinating after Hunter was born. An epidural may also cause your blood pressure to drop as blood vessels throughout your body relax. Before an epidural is placed you are "tanked up"—given fluid—and afterward your blood pressure is monitored frequently. If your blood pressure does drop, a small amount of ephedrine is given to bring it back up. This blood pressure lowering effect is temporary, although it may cause a transient drop in the baby's heart rate. If the baby's heart rate does drop, it invariably returns to normal within a minute or two as your blood pressure returns to normal. And, very rarely (about 1:1,000), the epidural needle may puncture the dura, allowing spinal fluid to leak out and causing a *spinal headache*. If this happens, lying flat in bed, pain medication, and caffeine usually take care of the headache; if not, a small amount of your blood is injected in the same spot, creating a patch—a blood Band-Aid—to prevent leakage. This blood patch is incredibly dramatic—one minute your head is exploding and the next you are up smiling.

Other than the potential for an epidural to cause a drop in your blood pressure, leading to a possible temporary drop in your baby's heart rate, an epidural has no impact on your baby. Nothing crosses the placenta. Babies are not depressed or drugged out—and neither are you. In my experience—both personally and professionally—moms who have epidurals give birth to wonderfully awake, alert babies.

I don't think any doctor—or nurse, or husband, or friend, or mother-in-law—should try to influence your decision about pain relief in labor. I think the people around you, including the medical staff, should support you in whatever you choose. I believe your doctor's job is to give you all the options but not to make the decision for you. As I tell all my patients, "I will tell you what your options are, the good and the bad points of these options, and I will support you if you want to avoid medication. I will not make these decisions for you because, after all, I am not in any pain when you are in labor!"

TABLE 38.1

Common Medications Used in Labor

Demerol (meperidine)
Narcotic. Probably the most commonly used narcotic in labor. Often combined with Phenergan to lessen the nausea Demerol often causes.

Inapsine (droperidol)
Another anti-nausea drug.

Morphine
Narcotic. Until Demerol's arrival in the 1940s, this was the most widely used narcotic for labor.

Nubain (nalbuphine)
This is a narcotic agonist-antagonist, meaning it has some narcotic properties, but in other areas it does not act like a narcotic. It tends to cause less nausea, and studies have shown it may work better in women than men, making it my favorite narcotic to use during labor.

Phenergan (promethazine)
A anti-nausea medication with sedative properties as well. Often given in conjunction with Demerol.

Stadol (butorphanol)
Another narcotic agonist-antagonist.

Zofran (ondansetron)
A powerful anti-nausea medication.

Frequently Asked Questions

Q After attending childbirth classes, reading, and talking to friends who have had babies, I'm pretty sure I'm going to want an epidural. Do I have to let anyone besides my doctor know my wishes, and how exactly is an epidural put in?

A *In addition to letting your doctor know now, be sure to tell the nursing staff when you are admitted to the hospital. The nurses will notify the anesthesiologist. Once you and your doctor decide it is an appropriate time to have an epidural, the anesthesiologist will talk to you about the benefits and risks of an epidural, and you will be asked to sign a consent form. By this time, you have had an IV started and will have gotten at least a liter of fluid. The anesthesiologist will have you get in the proper position. Some prefer you sitting, hunched over a pillow or table, while others prefer you lie on one side, knees curled toward chin, as much as a large pregnant belly will allow. This "cannonball" posture (think jumping off diving boards when you were 10) helps open up the spaces between the vertebrae, allowing the needle to be passed more easily. The anesthesiologist will then cleanse your back and numb the skin. A small introducer needle will be inserted between the vertebrae, with the smaller epidural needle passed through this. The doctor will feel a loss of resistance as the needle passes into the epidural space, and then he will thread a tiny catheter through the epidural needle and into this space. Before removing the needle, a test dose of medication will be given. Sometimes you may feel a twinge down one leg or another as the catheter is passed, and maybe a metallic taste in your mouth after the medication is injected. Once it is ascertained the catheter is in the correct location, the needle is removed and the catheter is taped to your back. You may be given a continuous low dose of medication, or you may be given intermittent doses when the effect of the first injection starts to wane. Once you deliver, the catheter will be pulled out. The entire process is pretty easy; the hardest part is holding still while you are contracting.*

Q I've heard an epidural can paralyze you. Is this true?

A *Do you live in the Philadelphia area? This was a common misperception when I was doing my residency at Temple University Hospital in Philly. Interestingly enough, it is not a comment I hear in my practice in Northern California! The answer is that you are not going to be paralyzed from an epidural. You may get a spinal headache if the needle is inserted too far, you may have a twinge down a leg as the catheter passes nerve roots, but you will not become paralyzed. A properly trained anesthesiologist or nurse anesthetist knows exactly where the needle needs to go, and the needle is neither large enough or sharp enough to sever your spinal cord, even if it is placed too deeply.*

Q I'm not sure whether I broke my water bag or not. I definitely did not have any floor-drenching gush, but my panties just seem continually damp. The baby is moving fine and I'm not having any contractions. What should I do?

A *Call your doctor and explain what you are feeling. If you were my patient, I'd have you come to the office or go to Labor and Delivery at the hospital (depending on the time of day that you call). Once there, an exam can be done to determine whether this is (1) ruptured membranes, (2) urinary leakage, (3) vaginal discharge, or (4) more moisture due to increased sweating. There are 2 basic ways to check for ruptured membranes. The simplest is to place a piece of nitrazine (pH) paper in your vagina; amniotic fluid (and blood) will turn the paper blue. The more precise way is to put a speculum into your vagina and collect any fluid or moisture present on a cotton swab. The swab is then smeared on a slide, which is examined under the microscope. Amniotic fluid dries in a characteristic pattern, like the fronds of a fern—hence the name fern test. If the nitrazine test is negative and no ferning is present, you did not break your water bag and you will be sent home.*

Week 39

SUN	DATE
MON	DATE
TUE	DATE
WED	DATE
THUR	DATE
FRI	DATE
SAT	DATE

What Happened This Week?

How I Feel Physically and Emotionally

Cesarean Section and VBAC

In the united States in 1999, 22 percent of all births were by cesarean section. The primary, or first-time c-section rate was 15.5 percent. Despite efforts to decrease the number of primary and repeat cesarean sections, the rate has gone up for 3 consecutive years, and the number of vaginal births after a previous cesarean (VBAC) has declined. However, whether this is really a bad thing is a matter of great debate in both ob-gyn and public health circles.

What Baby Is Doing

Your baby is ready and waiting to be born. Her grasp is firm and her limbs are flexed, "tiny knees curled to chin," as one of my daughter's favorite books (*On the Day You Were Born* by Debra Frasier, or according to Hunter, the "Born book, read Born, Mommy!") puts it. Her movements feel more like squirming (which is exactly what she is doing), as she no longer has much room for anything else.

Your baby is about 49 cm (19½ inches) and weighs 3,150 gm (6 lbs. 14 oz.).

What You Are Doing

You may notice a little bit of spotting after your doctor checks your cervix; this is normal and is nothing to be concerned about. You may be having trouble sleeping, both because you are getting up to urinate several times a night and because you are anxious about your baby's impending arrival. Swelling in your ankles and lower legs may be worse—be sure to report any other signs of pre-eclampsia (see week 34) to your doctor. If you are to have a cesarean section, it will be very soon, before you go into labor.

Special Considerations

Cesarean section rates are yet another thing that are higher in us over-35-year-olds. The overall c-section rate for a woman < 20 is 15 percent; for a woman > 40, it is almost 35 percent. Our higher rate of multiple births and complications like high blood pressure and diabetes is one reason for the higher chance of ending up with a cesarean. Another is that we may have already had one or more cesareans, and may choose a repeat c-section; after all, it is much more likely for a 35-year-old to be on her second or third pregnancy than would be an 18-year-old. But, even without a prior cesarean or any complications of pregnancy, you are still more likely to have a c-section, especially if this is your first child. Some doctors think of first-time pregnancies in older moms as "premium pregnancies," figuring it may have been difficult to get pregnant in the first place and there is less chance that you will be having more children after this. Because of this reasoning, some doctors are much quicker to reach for the scalpel with an older patient. I think this attitude is wrong. In my opinion, all pregnancies are premium, and the decision to proceed with a cesarean section should be made on firm medical ground—and the indications do not differ due to your chronological age.

What are some of the reasons a primary cesarean section may be necessary? The number one reason is *failure to progress,* a catch-all term meaning the baby got stuck somewhere in labor. Sometimes, labor is progressing slowly, you are getting frustrated, and so is your doctor; the quick—but not medically appropriate—remedy is to perform a c-section. Patience, perhaps some Pitocin, perhaps position changes or judicious use of pain medication may help you get over the hump and allow eventual vaginal delivery. Sometimes, even with intervention and assurance that your contractions are indeed strong enough (by placing an IUPC [intrauterine pressure catheter] to measure the exact strength of your contractions), you may not dilate beyond 4 or 6 or 8 centimeters. The baby's head may be just too big to fit through your pelvis (called *cephalopelvic disproportion,* or CPD); in this case, a c-section is the only way you will be able to deliver your baby. A few unfortunate women will become fully dilated and push, and push, and push, and push, but be unable to push the baby out—or to push him low enough so that the doctor can help out with a vacuum or forceps. This is called *arrest of descent.*

Another reason for a c-section is the baby being in a position other than head-down. Breech deliveries are more difficult than the usual vertex delivery, and risks to the baby are higher. Skill of the obstetrician is paramount in attempting a vaginal breech delivery—and because more and more breech babies are automatically delivered by cesarean section, fewer and fewer obstetricians possess these skills. Some doctors are not comfortable with attempting an external cephalic version either, one way of possibly lowering the number of cesareans due to breech position by turning these babies to the head-down position. The American College of Obstetricians and Gynecologists (ACOG) has published guidelines for attempted vaginal breech delivery, which include physician skills, the exact position of the baby (head flexed on chest, frank breech, which means the butt, rather than the feet, are first), and normal progression in labor. I—and most other obstetricians in private practice—have an additional criterion: you must have delivered a baby of at least roughly the same size vaginally before. If you've had a baby before, I know that you can get a baby through your pelvis and out your vagina. In a first-time mom, if I cannot successfully turn the baby with an external cephalic version, I will do a c-section.

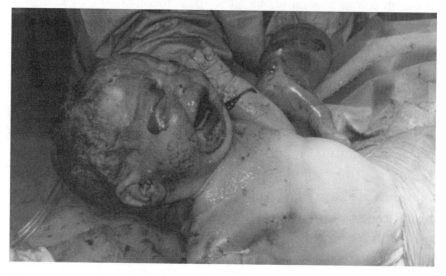

"Not-so-little Emma is delivered by repeat cesarean section. I'm easing her out of an incision in Kim's (age 40) lower abdomen. She looks like she'd rather stay where she was!"

The final significant reason for a c-section is fetal distress, another non-specific term for a heart-rate pattern the doctor is uncomfortable watching. True fetal distress, where the baby's heart rate bottoms out and will not come up with any intervention or where late decelerations happen contraction after contraction, does warrant an immediate c-section. Sometimes, the monitoring strip just doesn't look perfect, and labor is not progressing as rapidly as all would like, leading to a decision to perform a c-section before bad turns to worse. Despite all the c-sections for fetal distress, the incidence of *cerebral palsy* has not declined over the years; in fact, more and more evidence suggests that the events leading to cerebral palsy occur from chronic insults in the womb, long before labor begins.

Several other conditions can lead to a first-time cesarean. Virtually all triplets and higher are delivered via c-section, as are many sets of twins. If the lowest twin is head first, most of the time a vaginal delivery of both babies can be accomplished. If there is a placenta previa, a cesarean section must be performed; ideally, this is scheduled before you go into labor. A placental abruption, unless you are already pushing your baby out, will require immediate cesarean delivery, as will a prolapsed cord. A *prolapsed cord* means the umbilical cord drops out before the baby and can be compressed by the baby's head or body, cutting off the supply of oxygen and leading to fetal distress. Prior surgery on the uterus to remove fibroids (a *myomectomy*) may necessitate a c-section delivery, depending on how large the fibroid was and how extensive the incision into the uterine muscle was. Because a large, deep incision may weaken the muscle, causing the uterus to rupture during labor, a scheduled c-section is recommended in many cases. An active herpes outbreak when labor begins or the membranes rupture is an indication for a c-section, as is being HIV positive. In these cases, delivery by c-section markedly decreases the odds the infection will be passed to your baby.

In the United States, the largest category of c-sections are in women who have undergone one or more cesareans in the past. Until the 1980s, the saying was "once a cesarean, always a cesarean." Today, assuming the original incision on the uterus was low and horizontal (called a *low transverse* c-section), you will be offered the opportunity to choose a repeat c-section, scheduled several days prior to your due date, or an attempt at vaginal delivery. The latter is commonly referred to as a VBAC, for *Vaginal Birth After Cesarean*. Overall, about 70 percent of women attempting a VBAC will be successful, but that rate varies greatly depending on the reason for the original c-section. If you had a c-section the first time around because your baby was breech, and this one is head-first, your odds of a successful vaginal delivery are around 85 percent, just what they would be if you had never had a baby (or a c-section) before (remember, the first time c-section rate in the United States is 15.5 percent). On the other hand, if you pushed for 3½ hours last time, and then had a c-section, you only have a 12 percent chance of delivering vaginally.

Certain criteria must be met before you are considered a candidate for a VBAC. First, the scar on your uterus has to be transverse (side to side) and not vertical (up and down). A vertical scar is much weaker, because it goes right through the intensely contracting muscles, and the risk of uterine rupture during labor is 4–9 percent. With a transverse uterine scar, the risk of rupture is 0.2–1.5 percent (1 percent is the rate most commonly quoted). A uterine rupture is a catastrophic event that requires an immediate c-section for both your sake as well as that of your baby. For that reason, the second criteria for attempting a VBAC is that you labor in a hospital able to perform an emergency c-section immediately if a uterine rupture is suspected. Usually, if you have had more than two prior c-sections you will not be offered a VBAC, and some doctors will only offer a VBAC if you have had just one c-section in the past.

Your doctor has a responsibility to counsel you regarding the benefits (easier recovery, less blood loss, less chance of infection, shorter hospital stay) and risks (uterine rupture, which may be life threatening to you and your baby) of a VBAC. Your doctor has a responsibility to review your old records to ensure that you are indeed a candidate for VBAC, as the scar on your skin does not always mirror the scar on your uterus. Your doctor has a responsibility to give you at least some ballpark odds on success rates, given the review of why you had the first c-section. You have the responsibility of making the decision about whether you wish to try to deliver vaginally or to schedule a repeat c-section. The ultimate decision is yours, unless there is a medical reason like a prior vertical c-section, prior myomectomy, or this baby is breech, that you should not be allowed to labor. You should not feel pressured to choose one way or the other; you are not a wimp if you would rather know you are going to have your baby at 8 A.M. on the third Friday in November. You should not be coerced into attempting a VBAC, either. But if you choose a VBAC, your doctor should support that choice. In general, a woman who attempts to VBAC is treated like any other woman in labor—pain medications are given as needed and requested, and the delivery is exactly the same. The only differences are that continuous electronic monitoring of the baby is recommended if you are trying to VBAC (to pick up any early, subtle signs of uterine rupture) and that Cytotec (misoprostol) not be used to ripen the cervix.

If you do require (or choose, in the case of a scheduled repeat) a c-section, you can rest assured that this, the most common major surgery performed in the United States, is very safe for both you and your baby. Yes, there are risks, as there are with any surgery— and as there are with vaginal delivery—but major complications occur less than 3 percent of the time. An IV line will be started, and you will be given a liquid antacid to drink. You will be taken into the operating room, and, assuming this is not an emergency scenario, an epidural or a spinal will be administered. If it is an emergency, you will be put to sleep with general anesthesia. There will be a lot of people in the room: (1) the anesthesiologist at the head of the table; (2) your doctor and (3) an assistant to help with the surgery; (4) your labor nurse; and (5) perhaps a pediatrician; (6) a scrub nurse, to hand your doctor all the instruments; and (7) a circulating nurse, to get everything else everyone else needs. You will be positioned on the narrow operating table, with your arms extended at shoulder height, and you will be tilted a bit to your left to optimize blood flow to your baby (just like you didn't get to sleep on your back for all those months prior to today!). The top inch or so of your pubic hair will be clipped or shaved, and your belly will be cleansed with an antiseptic solution. Your bladder will be drained with a catheter, which will usually remain in place for 12–24 hours. Your doctor, who is scrubbed and ready to proceed, will lay a sterile drape across your belly, and will test to make sure the spinal or epidural has made you sufficiently numb. You should not feel any pain, but you will feel pressure and perhaps a tugging sensation as your baby is delivered.

Once you are "prepped and draped" and your support person is safely ensconced in a chair by your head, the actual surgery will begin. Your doctor will make a 6–8-inch cut about two finger-breadths above your pubic bone (in the bikini line), through the skin and all the underlying layers. A slightly smaller, transverse incision will be made on your uterus, and your baby's head (or butt, if he is breech) will be gently lifted out. The doctor will suction your baby's nose and mouth, and then she will deliver the rest of the body. The umbilical cord will be clamped and cut—your baby is born!—and he will be handed to a waiting nurse, to be bundled up and given to you to see and touch. All this takes less than 5 minutes (a bit longer if you've had a prior c-section due to scarring; that may take a couple of extra minutes to get through). Your doctor will then remove the placenta and gently swab your uterus to make sure all the membranes have been removed, then she will spend the next 15–20 minutes meticulously putting all the layers back together. She may close your skin with stainless steel staples (most common) or with a dissolvable suture just under the skin. Dressings are applied, you are transferred to a gurney and then to the recovery room. Soon, you will be in a postpartum room, able to snuggle with your beautiful new baby.

Frequently Asked Questions

Q I had a c-section with my first child, after getting stuck at 6 centimeters, and all my friends are pushing me to try a vaginal birth this time. I really don't want to; it was so hard to fail last time, and I don't think I can go through that again.

A *First of all, you are by no means a "failure" because you ended up with a c-section last time. The only "winning" in labor is having a healthy baby to take home—and it doesn't matter the path that baby took from your uterus to your arms! Second, who's having this baby anyway? You, or your friends? You. So, guess what, you make the choice that feels right to you. If that choice is to schedule a repeat c-section, great. If it is to try for a VBAC, well, that's great too. What is important is that you are given all the information you need to make the decision that is right for you—and everyone around you, from doctor to husband, from nursing staff to family and friends, should support you in that decision.*

Q I have had three children, all vaginally. But this time I'm carrying twins (yikes, 38 years old and about to have five children!), and the first baby is breech. I'm having a c-section next week. What can I expect from the recovery?

A *Expect your recovery from this c-section to be very different from that following a vaginal delivery. Your skin and all the layers underneath (fat, fascia, peritoneum, uterine wall) have been cut and sewn back together. Muscles have been stretched. You have undergone major abdominal surgery—and you have a new baby—no, two new babies!—to care for.*

You will have pain. It will hurt to stand up, it will hurt to roll over, and you will wonder how you will ever get out of your own bed at home, without the motorized adjustments. But, thanks to modern technology and the wonders of pharmacology, that pain is manageable. You may have gotten a narcotic through the spinal or epidural, which will make the first 24 hours almost pain-free. You may get a PCA (patient-controlled analgesic), a pump hooked up to your IV, through which you can give yourself a predetermined amount of narcotic whenever you need it. After the first 24–36 hours, you will be given oral pain medications to use as needed. Use them. Do not be a martyr.

The first few times you get up, you may feel as if your stitches are ripping apart. They are not. It is important to move about as soon as possible after surgery, to prevent pneumonia and blood clots and to help your intestines function properly. You will probably be given liquids right after the c-section, but solid foods may have to wait until you pass gas. You will stay in the hospital for 3–4 days after you deliver, assuming no complications.

Once you get home, you should have help. Heck, even if you had had a vaginal delivery you would need help caring for brand new twins, plus three other kids! I usually tell my patients: No lifting anything heavier than the baby. If you have stairs, for the first week or so, only go up and down them once or twice a day. I encourage walking on level ground—just to the mailbox at first, but gradually go farther and farther as you regain your strength. No housework! Let the dust bunnies fly, convince your husband that a vacuum is a power tool (well, it is!), or hire someone. Your older kids can help out—even my not-quite-2-year-old can wipe up spills on the floor. Don't expect to feel 100 percent in a couple of weeks—it will take 6–8 weeks to feel pretty good most of the time, and it may take longer to feel like your old self.

Q I had a c-section with my first baby because she was breech. This time, I plan on a vaginal delivery, but I want to give birth at home. My midwife says I will have to deliver at the hospital. What do you think?

A *I'm behind your midwife 100 percent. I'm not a big fan of home births in the first place, and a VBAC at home is a recipe for disaster. Only the lowest of low-risk women should even consider a home birth, and the fact that you have a scar on your uterus eliminates you from that low-risk category. Although the risk of uterine rupture dur-*

ing labor is only 1 percent with a transverse uterine scar, if a rupture occurs anyplace other than in a hospital capable of doing an immediate c-section, the overwhelming odds are that the baby will die—and you may die too. I am not trying to be dramatic or scare you, but just giving you the cold hard facts. Go for the VBAC attempt (you have about a 70 percent chance of success), but do it in the hospital, as your midwife quite correctly recommends.

Q I'd rather have a c-section than a vaginal delivery—I just don't want to deal with the pain of labor, or a stretched out vagina. My doctor says I can't have a c-section without a good reason. Why not?

A *A cesarean section is surgery, and all surgeries have risks. Yes, vaginal deliveries have risks too (and so does crossing the street), but those risks are not as great. With a c-section, blood loss is greater, the potential for needing a blood transfusion, while still low, is higher. Infection rates are much higher after c-sections than after vaginal births. There is also a risk of damaging the bladder during surgery.*

It is true that women who deliver vaginally are more likely to have problems down the road with urinary incontinence or uterine prolapse. Currently, there is a great debate in this country as to whether this possibility is great enough to justify purely elective c-sections, but as I write this, the answer is still "no".

Week 40

SUN   DATE

MON   DATE

TUE   DATE

WED   DATE

THUR   DATE

FRI   DATE

SAT   DATE

What Happened This Week?

How I Feel Physically and Emotionally

Labor Day

You have gotten through the days of endless retching and the nights of treks to the bathroom every half-hour. You have breathed through 6 weeks of childbirth classes. You have set up the crib and whittled the list of names down to a half-dozen finalists. Your bags are packed, the car seat is installed—Labor Day could be any day!

What Baby Is Doing

Your baby is getting pretty darn tired of the cramped quarters. His movements have slowed down in anticipation of birth (but if they stop altogether, call your doc right away!). His bowels are full of dark green-black meconium, the remnants of skin cells, amniotic fluid, and lanugo he has swallowed. If he has been stressed, he may pass some meconium before birth, but usually it is not eliminated until after delivery.

Both boys and girls have protruding breasts, thanks to the high levels of estrogen circulating in your blood stream. These will shrink in the few weeks after birth. For the same reason, girls may have some vaginal discharge, or even a small amount of vaginal bleeding.

At 40 weeks, your baby is about 50 cm (20 in) tall and weighs 3,400 gm (7 lbs. 7 oz.).

What You Are Doing

You are probably shifting in your chair trying to find a comfortable position as that bowling ball of a head presses on your bladder. You may have lost your mucus plug, and you may be having a slight blood-tinged discharge, especially if your doctor examined you recently. You may notice cramps radiating from back to front. You are about to make the transition from pregnant woman, a temporary 9-month condition, to mother, a lifelong state.

Special Considerations

If this is your first baby, you may wonder if you will know when labor begins. If this is not your first baby, you may still wonder the same thing! Those one in a million women whose babies fall out in the grocery store ("I just thought it was gas!") aside, I can tell you with confidence: You'll know. Imagine menstrual cramps. Now imagine them on steroids, coming every 5 minutes. I think you'll figure it out without too much trouble.

In general, you should call your doctor when your contractions are regular and uncomfortable. How far apart the contractions should be before you call depends on a lot of factors, including how far dilated you were at your last office visit; how far away from the hospital you live (a big factor where I practice, right up there with how much snow is on the roads!); how many children you have had before and how rapid (or slow) your previous labors were; and your own doctor's preferences. What I tell most of my patients (unless they live off the hill and it's winter) is to call when the contractions are every 5 minutes, they've been every 5 minutes for an hour and you want drugs! If your first two contractions are excruciating, then by all means call your doctor! If you live an hour away and delivered your first baby 10 minutes after you arrived at the hospital, then don't wait to call until you get the urge to push. Your doctor, who has examined you and who knows your circumstances, is the best person from whom to get explicit labor instructions.

When you arrive at the hospital, you will need to check in with the admissions office and from there will go to Labor and Delivery. If you are huffing and puffing, I can guarantee you will be wheeled as fast as possible to Labor and Delivery—admission clerks and ER docs do not want to have babies popping out in their departments, so if you feel you've been kept waiting a bit too long, just let out a moan! Once you arrive in the labor area, you will be asked to give a urine sample and will be placed on a fetal monitor. Your vital signs (temperature, pulse, and blood pressure) will be taken, and you will be asked several questions about your contractions, whether your membranes have ruptured, if you are having any bleeding or if you had any complications with your pregnancy. One of the labor room nurses (or residents—a doctor in training—if you will be delivering at a teaching hospital) will do an exam to determine if your membranes have ruptured and how far dilated you are. Don't expect your doctor to be there when you arrive, unless you told her on the phone you were bleeding heavily or had the urge to push. She will want to make sure it's the real thing before she (1) leaves her office, (2) leaves her dinner table, (3) leaves her child's piano recital, or (4) leaves her warm bed.

If you are not in "real" labor, you may be sent home, a frustrating but not uncommon scenario. It is better to wait for the real thing in the comfort of your own home than in the hospital. If you are in labor, you will be officially admitted. If your baby looks good on the initial monitoring, and if you want to, you can walk around or even take a nice warm shower. I encourage you to move about; not only does it feel better than lying in bed strapped to monitors, it allows gravity to help the course of labor.

Labor, by definition, means that you are having regular contractions that are causing your cervix to dilate and efface. There are three stages of labor:

1. **First stage.** This is broken into two phases, *latent phase* and *active phase*. The latent phase is early labor, when the contractions are regular, you may be effacing, but before there is much cervical change. This stage can last for many, many hours, but (fortunately) the contractions are not very intense. The active phase is characterized by progressive dilatation of the cervix, usually 1 cm/hr for a first timer and 2 cm/hr for a veteran. Some people consider active labor to begin around 3–4 centimeters. Although obstetrical textbooks do not recognize *transition* as a distinct phase of labor, this is a period when contractions are fast and furious, from 7–8 centimeters until you are fully dilated (10 cm).

2. **Second stage.** This begins when you are fully dilated and ends when your baby is delivered. This is the pushing stage. Pushing is where "labor" got its name—it is hard work. First-time moms push on average 50 minutes (with 3–4 hours of pushing not unheard of) and veterans for 20 minutes. Use of an epidural may increase these times, as it can be difficult to give it your all if you don't feel strong contractions or rectal pressure.

3. **Third stage.** This is the time from the delivery of your baby until the placenta is out. This is accomplished in a short amount of time, and with little or no effort on your part. Rarely, the placenta will not separate on its own and your doctor will have to reach inside your uterus to extract it.

If at all possible, try to stay home during the latent stage of labor. If your membranes have ruptured, you must call your doctor; the longer the membranes are ruptured, the greater the chance of

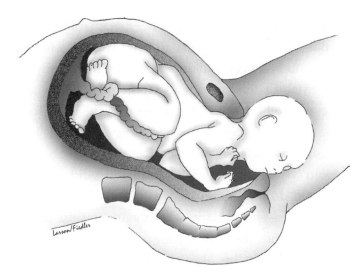

The moment of birth. Thanks to the hard work of pushing, the baby's head has emerged; once the shoulders are out, the rest of the body follows with little effort.

infection. In order to minimize the risk of infection to you and your baby, antibiotics are started 18 hours after rupture, sooner if your baby is preterm or if it is known you carry **GBS** (see week 31 Questions to learn more about GBS). If your membranes are intact, you can shower, take a warm bath (have help getting in and out of the tub!), walk, rest, and eat lightly until your contractions are more intense. I do not suggest foods like pizza or beef stroganoff—heavy and hard-to-digest foods may come back on you if you get nauseous later on!

Once you are in active labor, you will probably need to start practicing your relaxation techniques and breathing—or your use of the phrase, "I'd like an epidural now." Grabbing your partner's collar and screaming, "Get me drugs *now*," is also an effective technique. Your contractions are probably coming every 3–5 minutes, and may feel like squeezing a tube of toothpaste—if you imagine you're the paste! They often start at the top and move in a downward wave. You may have an increase in bloody show as you dilate and efface more. Your lower back may ache, especially if your baby is posterior, or nose pointing toward your belly, rather than toward your back. Firm pressure in your lower back (rolling pins, tennis balls, or your support person's fist all work well) can help with this backache. If you had been walking around quite happily until now, wondering what all this talk about labor hurting was about, you may notice yourself bent over, hanging on to the walls for dear life at this point—or you may calmly be telling yourself it is just your uterine muscle working as you visualize your cervix opening like a rose in bloom (visualization I tried, but that just didn't work for me).

Even if you do have an epidural, you will probably know you are 10 centimeters—fully dilated—before anyone else does. As your baby's head descends lower into your pelvis, you may notice a sensation or pressure, a feeling like you have to move your bowels. You may begin to involuntarily bear down. If I'm in a labor room and I hear grunting, I put gloves on! Many women feel an incredible sense of relief when they can begin pushing, saying it feels good to do something during the contractions. You can push squatting, lying on your side or semi-reclining, although at the very end, you will probably be asked to lie on your back, in that semi-reclining position, with your feet resting on supports or being held by your coaches. (I can't remember the last time I used the full leg stirrups, although I'm sure they are used in some places.) And, although I suppose some hospitals still take you back to a sterile delivery room, on a narrow metal table, to deliver, most deliveries in this country are done in birth rooms, in a birthing bed where the bottom can be removed for the actual delivery.

While you are pushing, your partner, the nurse, or your doctor may massage your perineum, helping it become more pliant and lessening the chance of your needing an episiotomy or tearing extensively. You may suddenly stop pushing effectively as the baby's head begins to crown, fearing the strange burning sensation at this point. Don't give up. "Push past the pain" is my mantra. This intense pressure and burning is your baby's head, stretching your perineum. This is the point where your doctor will cut an episiotomy if one is needed; if you do not have an epidural, your doctor will inject some lidocaine to numb the area before making the cut. A push or two more, your baby's head will emerge, your doctor will suction her tiny nose and mouth, a bit of a push for the shoulder, and then the rest of her wet, slippery body slides out, and your baby is placed on your chest. Congratulations, you did it. You are a mom! Get out the Kleenex as tears of joy flow. Don't be surprised if you see your doc wipe away a tear—no matter how many babies I deliver, each one is a miracle, and if Mom's crying and Dad's crying, well, count me in too!

After your beautiful baby is born, the doctor will cut—or will let your partner cut—the umbilical cord. Your precious bundle will be taken from you for just a minute, over to a warming bed to be dried off, have the umbilical cord re-clamped with a plastic clip, have identification bands put on, and be wrapped and brought back to you or another member of her fan club. Meanwhile, your doctor will obtain a tube of blood from the umbilical cord to check your baby's blood type and will deliver the placenta. If you had an episiotomy (or tear), it will be sutured. If you are planning to breastfeed, you can try right now—it also helps the placenta separate if it has not done so already.

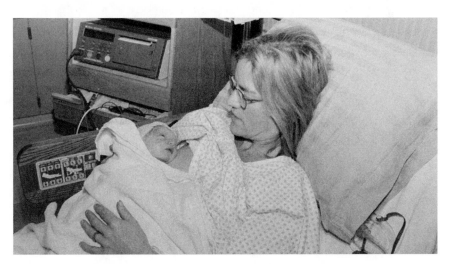

"Five minutes old. The expression on my face says it all: Now what do I do! Hunter, however, is possessed of the wisdom of the ages."

From My Journal

"12/3/98. Well, you arrived on 12/1/98 9:41 P.M. 5 lbs. 13 oz., 19 in long. I've been so busy staring at your beautiful face I haven't written anything until now. Here is the story of your birth:

We got to the hospital on 12/1 at 0630. Patty, the night nurse going off her shift put the first dose of cytotec in [my labor was induced]. I was 1/60/-2/V/I [translation: 1 cm dilated/60 percent effaced/head high/head first/membranes intact]. Mild contractions started pretty soon afterward, almost every 2 minutes. Jeff left to feed the dogs and do some work—besides, your dad does not do waiting well and I knew it could be a long day and night. I walked around, played Minesweeper on the nurses' computer—and won!—read, and was generally very comfortable. At 11, when Jan put in the second dose of cytotec, I was still 1 cm, but 80 percent effaced. Still very comfortable—you looked great on the monitor. I ate a veggie burger and took a nap. Lauren [my doc] checked me around 1 and I was 3–4 cm. By 3 P.M., I was starting to get more uncomfortable. Jeff came back and walked with me, rubbing my back during contractions. *Slow* progress—at 5 P.M. when Jan checked me again I was only 4–5, and I started thinking an epidural might not be such a bad idea! Lauren came in around 6 and said I was a tight 5 cm, so she ruptured my membranes and put in an IUPC [internal catheter to measure the strength of contractions]. It's amazing how warm amniotic fluid is! Then I realized the meaning of *pain*. Sheila came in to do the epidural. I sat up because I was more comfortable that way, but my intraspinous spaces were so tight she couldn't get the epidural in until she laid me on my side 45 minutes later—any other patient the anesthesiologist would have said, Tough, you're lying down. Oh well, sometimes it is not an advantage to be a doc because everyone kept asking what I wanted to do! I remember turning to Jan and saying, "I'm in transition and I'm losing it!" I think I said a certain four-letter word beginning with *s* a lot, too! Once the epidural was in, boy, did I feel better. I kept laughing and poking my legs because I couldn't feel them, although I could wiggle my toes. I think Jeff thought I was nuts, although he was also much happier—he didn't like seeing me in pain.

I think I got to fully dilated during the epidural, because I started feeling rectal pressure. I didn't say anything to Jan for a while, because I was enjoying being comfortable. When I did tell her I felt an urge to push, I was 10/+2! We waited for Lauren to arrive before I began pushing. You had some variables—head compressions—down to the 80s–90s, but with good recovery in between. It did scare me, though, and I told Lauren to go ahead and pull you out with the vacuum if she wanted, but about then you decided to behave, so I kept pushing. I pushed for 45 minutes, got a small episiotomy (at that point I didn't care), and watched in the mirror as your head emerged, followed by your tiny body. Jeff was too excited to cut the cord, so Lauren did—after a few whiffs of oxygen, Jan placed you on my chest, skin to skin. I put you to the breast and you latched on right away—thank God one of us knew what we were doing! You were incredibly alert and just looked around. There was the wisdom of the ages in your eyes. You were—and are—beautiful. 5 lbs. 13 oz. of miracle. We love you so much, Hunter Katherine Shanahan Turney."

Frequently Asked Questions

Q Because my baby is getting very big, my labor is going to be induced. What exactly does that entail? How will it feel different than natural labor?

A *There's more than one way to skin a cat—and to induce labor. If you are already 2–3 centimeters dilated, especially if you have already had children, your doctor may merely rupture membranes; this may be enough to get labor going. Pitocin, very similar to the oxytocin your body produces to make the uterus contract, is the most common agent used to induce labor. It is given through an IV drip. If your cervix is not very dilated or effaced, you may be brought in for "cervical ripening" first, a process in which a prostaglandin (usually Prepidil gel or a Cervidil suppository) is placed on or near your cervix in order to help it soften and thin out. Most of the time, Pitocin is begun after several hours to provoke regular contractions. A newer method of induction of labor is to use Cytotec (misoprostol), another prostaglandin. Although it is not FDA approved for inducing labor as a vaginal tablet, it is very effective, and Pitocin rarely has to be used.*

Pitocin usually accelerates and compresses the normal labor experience. Contractions can be strong from the get-go rather than building up more gradually. Exactly how the Pitocin is dosed is a big factor in this; if it is started at a very low dose and gradually increased, it is more like spontaneous labor. Many women, myself included, say that Cytotec induction is the closest thing you can get to a spontaneous labor experience, and are very happy with it. Frankly, since my induced labor was my only labor, I have nothing to compare it with, but I will take the word of my second- and third-time moms who have had spontaneous, Pitocin, and Cytotec labors!

Q What do you think about labor tubs and water birth?

A *I think laboring in water is a great idea, and would have done it myself had my hospital had a tub available. Because you can't be monitored while you are in the water, this option is limited to low-risk pregnancies, and ones in which initial monitoring is perfect. Another concern—and a possible reason why more hospitals don't have tubs— is the whole hygiene issue. There is potential for transmission of infectious agents in an improperly cleaned tub. While cleaning a regular bathtub is no big deal, sanitizing the intake pipes, jets, and other parts of a whirlpool tub is more involved. If a labor tub is not available, a warm shower can be very relaxing, too.*

Dr. Frederick Leboyer, author of Birth Without Violence, *first published in 1975, was a proponent of birthing in water. He—and many others—feel it is a less traumatic transition from the dark, watery womb to the outside world. With a water birth, you deliver in a tub, and then the baby is lifted from the water and placed on your chest, with his head out of the water. Babies will not take their first breath until they are brought into the air, so they won't drown. Water birth is more popular and widespread in Europe than it is in this country. Again, the hygiene issues probably will continue to limit its acceptance by the medical community. I have no experience with water birth, but if they made gloves that would cover me to my shoulders, I'd do a delivery this way.*

Q How will I know if my membranes rupture?

A *Most of the time, a woman knows when her membranes rupture. Sometimes there is a huge gush of fluid, so much that your shoes get wet. That is pretty hard to miss! Other times, there may be more subtle leaking, so that your panties are continually damp. Many women are unsure whether they had an accident or the water bag broke. When in doubt, call your doctor. She can do an exam to see if it is urine or amniotic fluid. You won't be bothering your doc—she'd be much more bothered if you didn't call, you got an infection, and you and your baby became sick as a result.*

Postpartum

SUN _____ DATE _____

MON _____ DATE _____

TUE _____ DATE _____

WED _____ DATE _____

THUR _____ DATE _____

FRI _____ DATE _____

SAT _____ DATE _____

_____

What Happened This Week?

_____

_____

_____

_____

How I Feel Physically and Emotionally

_____

_____

_____

_____

Postpartum: Where's the Instruction Manual?

CONGRATULATIONS! YOU DID it! Now, what exactly are you supposed to do with this tiny little bundle? First-time parents-to-be look at me as if I am nuts when I tell them pregnancy, labor, and delivery are the easy parts. Over the next days, weeks, and months, you and your baby will continue to go through some pretty amazing changes.

What Baby Is Doing

Eating, wetting, pooping, crying, and spitting up—that pretty much covers a newborn's repertoire. Oh, but don't forget looking absolutely angelic when she's sleeping. There are entire books about newborn care, and other than the fact that in December 1998 I actually took a baby home from the hospital, I am no expert—to paraphrase Butterfly McQueen in *Gone with the Wind*—and as I used to tell my patients, "I don't know nothin' 'bout taking care of no babies!"

Seriously, you've got to get a book (or if you are like me, a half-dozen) about caring for your new baby. Your little one is still developing. Her brain is growing, and new connections will form depending on the type of stimulation she receives now. Her digestive system is still figuring out what to do with that milk stuff your breasts or a bottle dutifully provide every 2–3 hours. She sees fuzzy shapes and can recognize a face. As many changes as there were from conception to delivery, there will be more over the next weeks, months, and years.

> ✎ DOCTOR'S NOTES
>
> Just a suggestion, from one mom to another: I kept a journal while I was pregnant (excerpts of which I've included throughout this book), but stopped after my daughter was born. Sure, I dutifully filled out the entries in the baby book and took untold rolls of pictures and videos, but I didn't record my feelings about sleep deprivation, or how I'd just stare for hours at her sleeping face—or how totally inept I felt at times. I regret not writing those things down. I hope you will keep a record of these first weeks and months, to pass on to your child someday.

What You Are Doing

If you had a vaginal delivery and an episiotomy, your perineum may be sore. Your upper back, neck, and shoulders may be sore, too, from pushing. If you had a cesarean section, your incision will hurt. You may be shocked the first time you stand up after having your baby—you still look about 20 weeks pregnant! Immediately after delivery, the top of your uterus is at your bellybutton; it will take 6 weeks for it to shrink back to its normal, pre-pregnancy size. This *involution* of the uterus is often accompanied by cramping, which tends to be more pronounced the more children you have had. Breastfeeding also accentuates this cramping, thanks to the natural hormone oxytocin involved in the milk let-down reflex. You may notice a slight increase in bleeding while nursing, too. Bleeding like a period lasts for 7–14 days, but *lochia,* a pinkish discharge that eventually becomes yellowish, can be present for 4–6 weeks. If you bleed heavily, soaking a maxi-pad in less than an hour for more than 1 hour, if your bleeding or discharge is foul-smelling, or if you have a fever, you should call your doctor.

If you are breastfeeding and you thought your breasts were big during pregnancy, just wait until your milk comes in! That can be good for another cup size. While small amounts of milk and colostrum are produced from the beginning, your full supply of milk does not come in until 3–4 days after birth. You may become engorged at first, until baby drinks his lunch, but the law of supply and demand will soon take effect, and your baby and your breasts will achieve a perfect balance. If you are not nursing, you should avoid any stimulation of your breasts and bind them with a firmly supportive bra. You can use cool compresses and take Tylenol to ease the discomfort that accompanies engorgement.

Special Considerations

"You're not really going to let us take this tiny, helpless baby home, are you?" were my thoughts as we prepared to leave the hospital 14 hours after I delivered. You have to get a license to drive a car, go through a federal background check to buy a gun, and be over 21 to buy a beer in many places, but absolutely anybody can have a baby and take him home, with no test to make sure they have the slightest clue about what to do with this vulnerable newborn. If you've never had a baby before, you may be thinking, "So, how hard can it be?" If my experience is any indication, it may be one of the hardest—and most rewarding—things you will ever do in your life.

Babies cry. A lot. They cry when they are hungry, when they are wet, when they want to be held, and when they just want you to leave them the heck alone. New moms cry, too. You cry because you are so tired (I used to be on call for 36 hours at a time, every third night, and that doesn't even begin to compare with the sleep deprivation of caring for a newborn!), because your hormones are on a roller coaster ride, because you don't know why the baby is crying, and because your baby is so beautiful you just can't believe it. Crying is a fact of parenthood. Knowing that does not make it any easier.

When your baby is crying and you are on the verge, it helps to have a systematic plan of attack. Eventually, if you follow the same steps every time, you'll find what it is your baby needs at that moment, and you will both stop crying. Here's what worked for me: (1) offer the breast or a bottle—this takes care of hunger, thirst, and the need to snuggle; (2) change the baby's diaper—they are almost constantly wet or poopy anyway; (3) put baby in the sling and walk around—movement is soothing to many newborns, who went everywhere with you for 40 weeks; (4) put baby down in her crib, just in case the baby really wants some quiet time—there is a lot going on in the world; newborns have an immature nervous system and it is easy for them to get overwhelmed; and (5) call for help. My husband could walk the floor for hours, or lie down with Hunter on his chest, and she'd drift off to sleep—not only are other people often better at calming babies than a wound-up mom, but it also gives you a break and makes the other person feel special and needed.

I remember a time when Hunter was about a month old; my mom, who had been here for 2 weeks, had left, and Jeff had gone back to work. I was nursing every 2–3 hours and trying to cook, clean the house, and keep up with my Internet work. I was exhausted and overwhelmed. Jeff came home to find me sitting at the top of the stairs, just crying. I was trying to do it all. I am not Superwoman, and neither are you. Superwoman is a comic strip character created by a man. You need help with a new baby. You need to learn how to ask for help and accept it when offered. I abdicated cleaning and food preparation, and was much happier. So what if we had pizza 3 nights a week—a vegetarian pizza has all the major food groups!

In retrospect, I can see that what I had was the baby blues, as do 70–80 percent of all new moms, or maybe even a mild case of postpartum depression. Some women (about 10 percent—not an insignificant number) have postpartum depression, with stronger feelings of sadness and anxiety. Women with postpartum depression may have trouble caring for themselves or their babies. Depression is more common in women with a prior history of depression or psychiatric illness, in women who do not have a supportive partner, or who live far from family or friends. It is not more common in us older moms, although I think if we have unrealistic expectations about caring for a newborn (as I did), you can set yourself up for depression. It is so easy when you are 38 and have excelled in your career to be overly critical of your "job performance" as a mother. The hormonal upheaval following childbirth is a powerful contributing factor; think PMS on steroids.

Postpartum depression can be treated. Most of the time, by just acknowledging it and asking for a little help from your loved ones, you will begin to feel better. If you talk to other new moms, you may not feel so alone—heck, if I had the blues, so can you. There is much to be said for the therapeutic benefit of a shower and wearing real clothes; if you haven't even taken 10 minutes a day for yourself to shower, you are likely to feel overwhelmed. I would put Hunter in a bouncy seat outside the shower door, so I could see and hear her while I luxuriated in the hot, hot water. Getting exercise and fresh air is good medicine as well. Sleep. When your baby is napping, you should too. Whatever you do, don't clean the house then! If you just aren't sleepy, read a couple of chapters in a novel, or paint your toenails fuchsia (hey, you can reach them again!), but don't do anything remotely resembling housework. If these suggestions don't help you combat the blues, call your doctor. She may suggest counseling or an antidepressant.

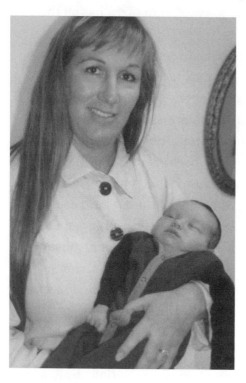

"Betty, age 41, is a pro holding two-week-old John, the latest addition to her family."

It took 40 weeks to grow your baby. It will take time for your body, your mind, and your spirit to return to "normal," too. You will never be the same person you were before becoming a mother, but you may be better. I know I am.

Frequently Asked Questions

Q My baby is 4 weeks old, and my doctor told me not to have sex until I was seen for the 6-week check-up. Do I really have to wait that long?

A *Some of your fellow new moms may be thinking, "Only six weeks? Maybe I can get my doctor to tell my husband he'll have to wait longer!" Everyone's sex drive is different, and while hormonal changes and exhaustion make many women feel like they'd be perfectly happy never having sex again, others like you are chomping at the bit. I would never countermand the advice of your own doctor, but I usually tell my patients nothing in the vagina for 4–6 weeks, or until all bleeding has stopped. If you have sex too soon, you may disrupt episiotomy stitches or increase the risk of infection if your cervix is still open. Before you light the candles and pull out a Victoria's Secret negligee, call your doc and ask her if it is okay if you have sex a little sooner than the 6-week mark.*

Q When I had the 2-week check-up after my c-section I forgot to ask my doctor about exercise. What can I do at this point?

A *You can walk. You can do Kegel exercises to tighten the vaginal muscles and minimize annoying postpartum incontinence (even with a c-section, the stresses of pregnancy alone may cause leakage of urine with coughing, sneezing, or laughing). You can push your baby in her stroller, on level and smooth ground. By the 4-week mark, you can go for longer walks, and may be able to ride a stationary bike. If you've stopped bleeding you can swim or do a water aerobics class. You can also do yoga. You should not do sit-ups or any weight lifting until your doctor specifically clears you for this. Living in the mountains, I tend to be more lenient than many doctors, allowing my patients to cross-country ski 3–4 weeks after a c-section and downhill ski or snowboard by 6 weeks (I cross-country skied about a week after my vaginal delivery, but I made my husband carry the baby!).*

Q I've been thinking about birth control—if I ever have sex again! I plan to breastfeed and I know that limits my options. What can I do to prevent back-to-back babies?

A *Actually, breastfeeding does not limit your contraceptive options very much at all. The only thing you can't use early on are combination oral contraceptives containing both estrogen and a progestin—the Pill, as we commonly think of it. Progestin-only pills (often called the mini-pill) like Micronor or Nor-QD are effective and do not interfere with your milk supply—or harm your nursing baby. DepoProvera and Norplant are two other progestin-only methods nursing moms can employ; DepoProvera is a shot given once every 3 months, and Norplant is a capsule placed in your upper arm, good for 5 years. You can use a diaphragm or a cervical cap, although if you have one from BB (Before Baby), you will need to be refitted at your 6-week check-up, because pregnancy changes you inside and out. Condoms are always an option, as is using a spermicidal gel, foam, film, or insert alone. An IUD is an attractive option for many women: IUDs are non-hormonal (the small amount of progesterone in the Progestasert IUD does not seem to affect anything other than the uterine lining), effective (99+ percent), and convenient (you don't have to remember to take a pill every day or interrupt foreplay to go find the darn diaphragm). Breastfeeding itself is fairly effective, but only for the first 6 months after delivery and only if you are nursing exclusively (no supplemental bottles or solid food) every 4 hours, around the clock.*

EPILOGUE

I'T'S FUNNY. As I typed the last word of the last chapter of this book, I had the same feeling I had after my daughter was born: a mix of pride and accomplishment, and a sense of sadness that the pregnancy (or in this case, the writing) was over. I have enjoyed writing this guide for you, as I enjoyed being pregnant. I hope you found it informative, and I hope my insights as both an obstetrician and an over-35 mom helped you get through the last 40 weeks. I wish you joy as you travel the lifelong road of motherhood.

Kelly

GLOSSARY

Abruptio placentae. See *placental abruption*.

Abruption. See *placental abruption*.

Active phase. The portion of labor beginning around 4 cm of dilatation and lasting until full dilation at 10 cm.

AFP. See *alpha fetoprotein*.

Afterbirth. Another name for the placenta.

Afterbirth pains. Cramping after delivery, due to involution, or shrinkage, of the uterus.

Air embolism. Entry of air into blood vessels that leads to obstruction of the vessel. If this lodges in the lungs, oxygen cannot enter the blood stream; large embolisms can be fatal.

Alpha fetoprotein. A protein produced by the baby and present in amniotic fluid and maternal blood. Elevated in neural tube and abdominal wall defects. Commonly abbreviated AFP.

Alveoli. Thin-walled sac at the end of the respiratory tree. Gas exchange between the air you breathe and blood in capillaries occurs here.

Amniocentesis. Removal of amniotic fluid from around the baby. Often used to determine the baby's chromosomal makeup. Also may be done to check for lung maturity or infection.

Amnion. Innermost membrane of the amniotic sac surrounding the amniotic cavity.

Amniotic cavity. Fluid-filled space which contains the baby and the placenta.

Androgen. Male hormone. Hormones like testosterone that encourage development of male sex characteristics.

Anemia. Low red blood count. May contribute to fatigue.

Anencephaly. Birth defect in which the skull and brain do not develop properly; anencephaly is incompatible with life.

Antenatal testing. Ways of evaluating the health of the baby before birth. *Includes non-stress tests, contraction stress tests, and biophysical profile.*

Antibody. An immune molecule that reacts with a specific antigen. Antibodies can confer immunity to certain infections and are the basis for immunizations.

Antigens. Substances that induce an immune response.

Aorta. The large artery that takes blood from the heart to the rest of the body.

Apnea. Lack of breathing.

Areola. Pigmented area surrounding the nipple.

Arrest of descent. The baby's head becomes "stuck" after full dilation. Inability to push the baby out or deliver vaginally after becoming fully dilated.

Bacterial vaginosis. AKA Gardnerella, a bacterial infection which may cause a malodorous, painful vaginal discharge. There is some evidence that bacterial vaginosis may increase the risk of preterm labor.

Betamethasone. A steroid given to enhance lung maturity in cases of preterm labor.

Bimanual examination. Examination of the uterus and ovaries accomplished by the doctor placing one gloved hand in the vagina and the other on the lower abdomen.

Biophysical profile. A type of antenatal testing composed of an ultrasound to evaluate the baby's activity and a non-stress test.

Biparietal diameter. The greatest transverse diameter of the head, roughly from ear to ear. Commonly abbreviated BPD, it is an ultrasound measurement used to estimate the baby's age.

Blastocyst. Ball of blastomeres with a central fluid-filled cavity. Begins once there are 50–60 blastomeres. It is at this stage that implantation occurs.

Blastomere. One of the cells into which the egg divides after fertilization. These cells have the potential to become any cell type or body part.

BPD. See *biparietal diameter.*

Bradycardia. Slow heart rate. Prior to birth, a heart rate of <100 bpm as determined on fetal monitoring.

Braxton Hicks contractions. Irregular, mild contractions that do not cause the cervix to dilate.

Breech. Buttocks, or a baby that is butt down.

Brethine. Brand name for terbutaline, which can be used to stop contractions leading to premature labor.

Bronchi. The two main branches of the trachea, conveying air to the lungs.

Bronchioles. Smaller branches off the two main bronchi; there are approximately six increasingly fine divisions terminating in the aveoli.

Bronchopulmonary dysplasia. Scarring of the bronchi and lungs, usually as a result of extreme prematurity and need for mechanical ventilation, that impairs lung function.

Brown fat. Fat that helps with heat production after birth.

Capacitation. Process in which proteins are removed from the head of a sperm, allowing it to penetrate and fertilize an egg.

CBC. Complete blood count. Measures white blood count (indication of infection) as well as hemoglobin and hematocrit (markers for anemia).

Cephalopelvic disproportion. The baby's head is too large to fit through mom's pelvis.

Cerclage. Stitch placed in an incompetent cervix to prevent premature dilatation and loss of the baby.

Cerebral palsy. Brain injury, usually occurring before birth or during labor, that can lead to problems with coordination, walking and other muscle function. Sometimes associated with mental retardation.

Chlamydia. Sexually transmitted disease caused by Chlamydia trachomatis, which may have no symptoms in women and may lead to blockage of the tubes.

Chloasma. Irregular patches of brown pigment on the face. Also called the "mask of pregnancy," this is stimulated by pregnancy hormones increasing melanin pigment in the skin.

Chorion. Outermost membrane forming the amniotic sac surrounding the amniotic cavity.

Chorionic villus sampling. Biopsy of the developing placenta in order to perform genetic testing.

Chromosomes. Object within the nucleus of the cell that contains our genes. There are 46 chromosomes in humans, arranged in 23 pairs—one from mom and one from dad.

Clomid. Brand name of clomiphene citrate.

Clomiphene. An estrogen-like drug that is used to induce ovulation.

CMV. Cytomegalovirus. A viral infection, common in young children.

Collagen. A protein comprising connective tissue in the body.

Colostrum. First milk, high in antibodies which confer immunity to the newborn during breastfeeding.

Contraction stress test. A type of antenatal testing in which contractions are provoked and the baby's response to them is monitored.

Cord accident. Acute problem of the umbilical cord such as a knot, prolapse or coiling around a body part that cuts off blood supply to the baby.

Corpus luteum. Cyst on the ovary that produces progesterone after ovulation.

Cortisol. A steroid hormone.

CPD. See *cephalopelvic disproportion.*

CRL. See *crown-rump length.*

Crown–rump length. Measurement from the top of the baby's head to its buttocks. Done via ultrasound to determine the baby's age.

CST. See *contraction stress test.*

Cunnilingus. Oral sex performed on a woman.

CVS. See *chorionic villus sampling.*

D&C. Dilatation and Curretage. A minor surgical procedure to dilate the cervix and remove the contents of the uterus. May be done to complete a miscarriage, perform an elective abortion or remove an adherent placenta after delivery.

Decelerations. Drops in the baby's heart rate. May be **early,** due to head compression; **late,** due to placental insufficiency; or **variable,** due to cord compression.

Decidual reaction. Thickening and increased secretions of the uterine lining in response to pregnancy.

Deciduous teeth. Non-permanent teeth; baby teeth.

Diastasis rectii. Separation of the paired abdominal muscles (rectus muscles) that run from the breastbone to the pubic bone as a result of the enlarging uterus.

Dizygotic twins. Fraternal (non-identical) twins arising from fertilization of two different eggs by two different sperm.

Doppler flow study. A type of antenatal testing in which blood flow through the umbilical cord is measured.

Doppler. Hand-held device used to listen to the baby's heartbeat.

Down syndrome. Genetic defect caused by an extra chromosome 21. Also called *Trisomy 21,* it is associated with varying degrees of mental retardation and physical defects.

Ductus arteriosis. Connection between the pulmonary artery and the aorta that allows most blood to bypass the baby's non-functional lungs.

Duodenal atresia. Absence or constriction of the junction between the stomach and the small intestine.

Eclampsia. Seizures as a consequence of uncontrolled *pre-eclampsia.*

Ectoderm. Outer layer of the embryonic disc that will give rise to skin, hair, and the nervous system.

Ectopic pregnancy. Pregnancy that develops outside the uterus, most commonly in a fallopian tube.

EDC. Estimated date of confinement. The due date, calculated as 280 days from the first day of the last menstrual period.

Effacement. Thinning of the cervix.

Embryo. The baby from weeks 4–10.

Embryonic disc. Collection of cells at one end of the blastocyst that will form the baby.

Endoderm. Inner layer of the embryonic disc that will give rise to the lungs and digestive system.

Endometrium. Uterine lining

Engagement. The baby's head (or breech) enters the pelvis.

Epicanthal folds. Tissue at the inner corner of the eye.

Epidermal ridges. Ridges on the palms of the hands and soles of the feet that are the basis for fingerprints.

Esophageal atresia. Absence or narrowing of the junction between the esophagus (swallowing tube) and the stomach.

Estrogen. Female hormone.

Exchange transfusion. Blood transfusion in which some of the recipients blood is withdrawn to make room for transfused blood. Done in cases of sickle cell anemia and in extreme newborn jaundice.

Fellatio. Oral sex performed on a man.

Fern test. A way to diagnose ruptured membranes; amniotic fluid, when dried on a slide, will form a fern-like pattern.

Fetus. The baby from 10 weeks until birth.

Fibroid. A benign growth of the uterine wall muscle.

FISH. Fluorescent in-situ hybridization. A technique to rapidly identify chromosomal abnormalities in amniocentesis or CVS specimens. Most often used to look for Trisomy 18, Trisomy 21 (Down syndrome) and Fragile X.

Folate. Another name for folic acid.

Folic acid. One of the B vitamins, adequate levels of folic acid at the time of conception decrease the odds of a neural tube defect.

Follicle. A developing egg.

Fraternal twins. See *dizygotic twins*.

FSH. Follicle stimulating hormone. Stimulates egg development.

Gardnerella. See *bacterial vaginosis*.

GBS. See *Group B strep*.

Geneticist. A specialist in the diagnosis of and counseling regarding genetic (inherited or chromosomal) disorders.

Gestational diabetes. Abnormal glucose metabolism (diabetes) that develops only during pregnancy.

Gestational sac. An early pregnancy, visible on vaginal ultrasound by 4 weeks.

Glucola. Special glucose drink used in glucose tolerance tests.

Glucometer. Device for measuring blood sugar using a drop of blood from a finger stick and a special hand-held monitor.

Glucose tolerance test. Test to measure the body's response to a glucose (sugar) load. Blood sugar levels are drawn at predetermined intervals following a glucose drink.

Glycosylated hemoglobin. Hemoglobin to which glucose is attached. Serves as a measure of sugar control in diabetes.

Gonadotropins. Hormones, produced in the brain, that stimulate ovarian function.

Gonorrhea. Sexually transmitted disease caused by Neisseria gonorrhea, producing a yellow, pus-like cervical discharge.

Gravida. Number of pregnancies, including the current one.

Group B strep. A strain of the streptococcus bacteria.

HCG. Human chorionic gonadotropin, the pregnancy hormone secreted by the baby.

HELLP syndrome. Severe pre-elampsia complicated by abnormalities in the liver and blood clotting systems.

Hemoglobin. Oxygen-carrying pigment in red blood cells. Used as a measure of anemia.

Hydrocephalus. Excess fluid in the brain. Also called "water on the brain."

Hydronephrosis. Dilation of a kidney due to partial or complete blockage of a ureter.

Hyperemesis gravidarum. Excessive vomiting during pregnancy leading to dehydration and malnutrition.

Identical twins. See *monozygotic twins*.

In vitro fertilization. A technique to fertilize the eggs outside the body and return the embryo(s) to the uterus. So called "test tube baby" technique.

Incompetent cervix. Cervix that is weak and dilates without contractions. May lead to a second trimester miscarriage or premature birth.

Insulin. A peptide hormone produced in the pancreas that regulates blood sugar levels.

Intrauterine growth restriction. Poor growth of the baby, often leading to a low birthweight baby.

Intraventricular hemorrhage. Bleeding into the brain, usually in extreme prematurity.

Intubation. Process of placing a breathing tube; once the breathing tube is placed, one is intubated.

Involution. Return of the enlarged uterus to its normal size after pregnancy.

IUGR. See *intrauterine growth restriction.*

IUPC. Intrauterine pressure catheter. A slim tube inserted into the uterus through the dilated cervix in order to directly measure the strength and duration of contractions.

IVF. See *in vitro fertilization.*

IVH. See *intraventricular hemorrhage.*

Kegel exercises. Exercises to tighten the vaginal and pelvic floor muscles.

Ketones. A substance, like acetone, produced by carbohydrate and fat metabolism in times of starvation.

Ketosis. Increased production of ketones during times of starvation or in poorly controlled diabetes.

Kick count. A type of antenatal testing in which the number of times the baby moves is recorded.

Lanugo. Soft, downy, pale hair covering the baby's body.

Latent phase. The earliest stages of labor, prior to 4 cm.

Level II ultrasound. See *targeted ultrasound.*

LGA. Large for gestational age. A big baby.

LH. Luteinizing hormone. Secreted in the brain, LH is vital in final ripening of the follicle and ovulation.

Linea nigra. Pigmented line down the center of the abdomen.

Listeria monocytogenes. Bacteria found in many sources, including soft cheeses.

LMP. Last menstrual period. By convention, indicates the first day of the last period.

Lochia. Discharge of blood, mucus and debris after childbirth. Intially red (lochia rubra) it becomes yellow-white after several weeks (lochia alba).

Low birthweight. Weight less than 2500 gms (5 lbs 7 oz).

Lumbar lordosis. Exaggerated inward curving of the lower back during pregnancy. Swayback.

Luteal phase defect. Low levels of progesterone after ovulation. May contribute to some cases of miscarriage.

Macrosomia. Large baby, often the consequence of uncontrolled diabetes.

Mesoderm. Middle layer of the embryonic disc that gives rise to the bones, muscles, reproductive and circulatory systems.

Methotrexate. A folic acid antagonist, it can be used to medically dissolve ectopic pregnancies.

Miscarriage. Spontaneous loss of the baby in the first 20 weeks of pregnancy.

Missed abortion. Nonviable pregnancy that does not immediately miscarry. The traditional definition requires that the baby be dead at least 4 weeks, but with advent of ultrasound, now refers to any unsuccessful pregnancy before the onset of cramping or bleeding or passage of tissue.

Monochorionic. In a twin pregnancy, instead of the normal two layers of chorion in the dividing membrane, there is only one. Found in monozygotic twins.

Monozygotic twins. Identical twins, formed from one fertilized egg that divides into two separate beings early in pregnancy.

Morbidity. The rate of illness or complications.

Mortality. The rate of death.

Morula. A solid ball of blastomeres.

NEC. See *necrotizing enterocolitis.*

Necrotizing enterocolitis. Inflammation of the bowel wall.

Neonatologist. A pediatrician who specializes in care of premature and sick babies.

Neural groove. Initial indentation down the baby's back that will later fold over to form the neural tube.

Neural tube defects. Incomplete closure of the neural tube leading to *spina bifida* or *anencephaly.*

Neural tube. Hollow tube of cells along the baby's back that will become the spinal cord and brain..

NICU. Neonatal intensive care unit. Specialized nursery to care of very premature or sick newborns.

Non-stress test. A type of antenatal testing in which the baby's heart rate is monitored and recorded on a paper tracing.

NST. See *non-stress test.*

Nuchal cord. A loop of umbilical cord wrapped around the baby's neck.

Oligohydramnios. Less than the normal amount of amniotic fluid.

Omphalocele. Herniation of intestines or other abdominal contents into the base of the umbilical cord.

Organogenesis. Development of all the major organ systems during the embryonic period.

Parity. Number of previous deliveries, excluding miscarriage, abortion, or ectopic pregnancy.

PDA. Patent ductus areriosis. Lack of closure of the ductus arteriosis after birth.

Pelvic rest. Avoidance of anything placed into the vagina.

Pergonal. A gonadotropin medication used to induce ovulation.

Perinatologist. An obstetrician who has additional training, specializing in the care of high-risk pregnancies.

Perinuem. The skin and underlying tissues between the vagina and rectum.

Placenta accreta. Placenta that is abnormally adherent to the uterine wall.

Placenta increta. Some of the placenta invades the uterine wall muscle.

Placenta percreta. Part of the placenta penetrates the full thickness of the uterine wall and may actually invade adjacent organs like the bladder.

Placenta previa. Part or all of the placenta covers the cervix.

Placental abruption. Separation of part or all of the placenta from the wall of the uterus prior to delivery of the baby.

Polyhydramnios. Excessive amniotic fluid.

Pre-eclampsia. High blood pressure and *proteinuria* complicating pregnancy.

Progesterone. Steroid hormone produced by the corpus luteum and the placenta.

Proteinuria. Protein in the urine.

Pulmonary edema. Fluid in the lungs, interfering with breathing and oxygenation.

Quickening. First sensation of feeling the baby move.

RDS. See *respiratory distress syndrome*.

REM sleep. Period of rapid eye movement, associated with dreaming.

Respiratory distress syndrome. Difficulty breathing due to immature lungs.

Restless leg. Spasms of calf muscles leading to uncomfortable leg twitches shortly after falling asleep.

Retinopathy of prematurity. Eye damage in premature babies due to abnormal growth of blood vessels.

Rh factor. A blood group antigen. If you have the factor, one is Rh postive, but if you lack it, you are Rh negative.

RhoGAM. An immune globulin given to prevent formation of anti-bodies to the Rh factor in women who are Rh negative.

Ritodrine. A medication given to stop contractions. A tocolytic.

Round ligament. Ligaments that stretch from near the top of the uterus to the pelvic side wall.

RPR. A test for syphilis.

Rubella. AKA German measles, caused by a virus, which produces a red rash and enlarged lymph nodes.

S<D. Size less than dates, meaning the uterus is smaller than expected.

S>D. Size greater than dates, indicating the size of the uterus is bigger than the gestational age would suggest.

Sciatica. Pain in the buttocks and back of the leg caused by compression of the sciatic nerve.

SGA. Small for gestational age. A small baby, but not necessarily low birthweight.

Shoulder dystocia. Entrapment of the shoulders following delivery of the head.

Somites. Bundles of mesodermal cells paired on either side of the neural groove that will give rise to the vertebra.

Spina bifida. A *neural tube defect* caused by incomplete closure of the lower spine. Depending on the degree of exposed spinal cord, spina bifida may be associated with paralysis of the legs and *hydrocephalus*.

Spinal headache. Headache caused by escape of spinal fluid. Occurs after a spinal anesthetic or an epidural which inadvertently punctured the dura.

Stress incontinence. Involuntary leakage of urine associated with coughing, sneezing, laughing, or other activities.

Surfactant. Substance forming a film over the alveoli that prevent them from collapsing during breathing.

Sutures. Membranous connections between the various bones of the skull.

Syphilis. A sexually transmitted disease caused by a spirochete (Treponema pallidum) which may produce a genital ulcer. If untreated, it may involve the heart and brain.

Tachycardia. Rapid heart rate. In babies, greater than 160 bpm.

Targeted ultrasound. An ultrasound to look for structural birth defects. More comprehensive and detailed than a regular ultrasound, and usually performed under the auspices of a perinatologist.

Teratogens. Any substance or agent that can cause abnormal fetal development.

Terbutaline. A tocolytic medication. The generic name for Brethine.

Tocolytic. A medication which stops uterine contractions.

Toxoplasmosis. Disease caused by a parasite found in cat feces and undercooked meats.

Transition. Stage of labor immediately preceding full dilatation.

Triple screen. A blood test which includes AFP, HCG and estriol, and is used as a screening test for neural tube defects, Down syndrome and Trisomy 18.

Trisomy 18. An extra copy of chromosome 18.

Trisomy 21. See *Down syndrome.*

Trophoblasts. Outer layer of cells on the blastocyst which invade the uterine lining and eventually form the placenta.

Tuberculosis. Lung infection caused by Mycobacterium tuberculosis.

Ultrasound. High frequency sound waves that when bounced off a structure (like a baby) produce an image on a screen.

Ureter. Tube that travels along the pelvic side wall, draining urine from the kidney into the bladder.

VBAC. Vaginal birth after a prior cesarean section, or the attempt thereof.

Vena cava. Large vein returning blood from the lower body back to the heart.

Vertex. Head. Usually refers to the baby being head first.

Viability. Ability to survive on one's own, outside the uterus.

White fat. Fat important in energy storage.

Yolk sac. Small round rim of cells that provide nutrients and blood cells for the early embryo.

Zygote. The baby from fertilization until the beginning of the embryonic period.

INDEX